PMS

PMS

What It Is and What You Can Do About It

Sharon M. Sneed, Ph. D.
and
Joe S. McIlhaney, Jr., M.D.

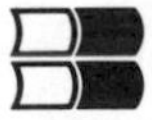

BAKER BOOK HOUSE
Grand Rapids, Michigan 49516

ISBN: 0-8010-8290-0

Sixth printing, September 1989

Printed in the United States of America

Contents

Part Four Living with PMS

Introduction

I [Sharon] am one of you. I spent years of my life not knowing why I had strange feelings at various times of the month. I spent sleepless nights wondering about intermittent aches and pains. I anguished over unfortunate words spoken to a child, knowing that I was temporarily out of control and overwhelmed with tension and irritability.

I am also a research scientist and have worked for years in a laboratory learning to be objective. From observations of myself and other patients, I am convinced that PMS is absolutely real. I am equally convinced that treatment makes a difference.

If you, too, suffer from PMS, you may be unhappy with yourself and your behavior toward others, and wonder if there is any way to correct your situation. Read on. Diagnosis and treatment are within reach.

During the week prior to your menstrual period:

1. Do you feel more irritable than usual?
2. Is your efficiency diminished?
3. Do you have food cravings and an increased appetite?

4. Does your mood change suddenly, usually without apparent reason?
5. Do you gain weight?
6. Do you have insomnia or feel unusually fatigued?
7. Do you have headaches?
8. Do you doubt your judgment or have trouble making decisions?
9. Do you have breast tenderness?
10. Is there a change in your sexual behavior?

If you answered "yes" to even a few of these questions, you may have what has become known as the premenstrual syndrome (PMS). Don't be surprised at this possibility, though. It is estimated that 90 percent of all women have some degree of premenstrual tension, and probably one-third of all menstruating women have a full-blown case of PMS, complete with many of the symptoms listed in the questions above.

As practicing clinicians who have helped numerous PMS patients, we firmly believe that treatment is crucial. It can literally change your life—your outlook, your productivity, your relationships with others.

As Christians, we recognize that treatment is also crucial for your spiritual life. In this book, we stress the fact that PMS is not a spiritual problem. However, there is usually so much anxiety and tension accompanying PMS that many Christians equate its symptoms with a weakened relationship with God. We do not agree with this association.

We do feel that proper treatment will allow you to be your "normal" self all or most of the time. This is so much better for your general sense of well-being than behavior that swings like a pendulum between the "normal you" and the "PMS you."

Who Needs to Read This Book?

Women with PMS

You know who you are already or you would probably not be reading this now. Our goal in writing this book is to provide you with a step-by-step guide for both self-treatment and professional help. If you are diagnosed as having premenstrual syndrome, first of all, accept the reality of PMS—don't deny its existence. Second, accept the responsibility of PMS—don't neglect treatment.

Spouses of Women with PMS

An understanding husband can be a great asset for a woman with PMS. A husband whose wife has severe PMS problems may be at his limit of tolerance. Understanding a wife's problem is the first step toward extending that tolerance. Helping her with her own treatment program is the next move. This book will help husbands to accomplish both of these goals.

Children, Parents, and Workmates of Women with PMS

The woman herself must be the judge about which of her friends and relatives need an understanding of her PMS problems. If you have PMS, depending on the ages of your children, you may want to explain things to them—especially if your behavior has caused rifts and stresses in your relationship in the past. (PMS has been listed as a significant contributing factor of child abuse.) The quality and circumstances of other relationships (relatives, friends, co-workers) will determine who might benefit from understanding PMS, especially as it relates to your situation.

This Is a Handbook

This book includes many suggestions for you to actively participate in setting up your own treatment program.

Also provided are flow charts and summaries of various treatment options, including:

Advice on choosing a physician
The PMS diet program
Importance of the PMS calendar
The PMS exercise program
Drugs, vitamins, and minerals used in PMS treatment

With this book, you may be able to solve PMS with self-help only. If you need further help, we have provided the guidelines for what to expect when seeking professional assistance. This information should aid you in choosing the right physician and in asking informed questions.

Part 1

Recognizing PMS

1

Sharon's Story

I'm really not sure when the words *premenstrual tension* became known to me. It definitely wasn't during my teenage years. We barely even discussed the issue of menstruation at home, probably because it was considered an unmentionable though necessary bodily function. In junior and senior high school it wasn't a big topic of conversation either, even among my friends. In fact, my only recollection of our taking note of menstruation was in junior-high gym class. But the menstrual cycle was not openly or positively discussed. Rather, it remained a somewhat murky subject that could elicit feelings ranging from intolerable embarrassment to pride and enviability, depending on who was listening.

Of my high-school years, I have some wonderful memories of seemingly endless and happy times, but I also recall some very difficult days. Sounds typical of the teen years, doesn't it? In retrospect, however, I believe that my own PMS symptomology could have begun during that time. There are vague remembrances of days when my classes went well, exam grades were good, and I had a weekend date to look forward to (all the important things to a seventeen-year-old). Yet even then I had an uneasy feeling that something was not quite right. Feelings of anxiety over insignificant issues were common during certain "bad days." Emotional outbursts within my nuclear family and feelings of low self-esteem sometimes spoiled things for me. I can also remember that what should have been relatively small problems sometimes loomed as major tragedies. My recall of events is not so complete as to allow a direct correlation between those tough days and premenstrual tension, and I'm sure that some of those reactions were merely "normal" teenage behavior (whatever that may be). In short, because I had little, if any, knowledge of PMS symptomology through high school and even my undergraduate college days, I never entertained the idea that my sporadic anxieties might be cyclical in nature. However, my suspicion is that many of these unpleasant memories were PMS-related because they seemed to just come and go with no apparent underlying reason. Several health professionals have recently proposed that PMS does begin in the teen years.

At age twenty-one, I married and began taking an oral contraceptive. This was really the time when my premenstrual tensions began to worsen. Thinking that my vague and intermittent anxieties revolved around "newlywed adjustment," I ignored many of the definite mental and physical signs—water retention, inordinate fatigue, headaches, inability to concentrate, depression, decreased sexual drive—and supposed that I just didn't like marriage as much as I thought I would. When I stopped the oral contraceptives four years later, I can still remember that these problems seemed to diminish. It seemed such a remarkable difference, in fact, that I distinctly remember mentioning it to my sister, who spontaneously replied that she had experienced the same feelings when she stopped taking oral contraceptives. I am now aware that for some women oral contraceptives can intensify PMS problems, though for others it may actually alleviate the symptomology. It also stands to reason that my biologic sister might have PMS problems similar to my own, since it has become clear that PMS is, to a certain extent, a genetically determined trait.

When my husband and I began working on a family one year later, we were stunned when our first two pregnancies ended in miscarriage. Following this, we had a full-term, healthy baby, followed by two more miscarriages and then the birth of two more healthy babies. My physicians could give no explanation for the miscarriages (spontaneous abortions), but hormonal imbalance in the first trimester was certainly a major suspect. I am now aware that miscarriages may be more common with women who experience some of the more severe symptoms of premenstrual syndrome. Also typical of PMS women, I experienced a great euphoria in the last half of my full-term pregnancies and a rather severe postpartum depression after the end of breastfeeding these babies (this coincides with the onset of periods again, after both the pregnancy and the breastfeeding have stopped). I wish that I had known then what I know now about PMS. At the time, I was intolerant of my postpartum depression, even feeling guilty about my thoughts. I considered myself ungrateful, weak-willed, and perhaps even mentally unstable for having these feelings of anxiety at a time that should have been filled with joy over a new birth. If someone could have told me that I was experiencing classical PMS-related postpartum anxieties, I think that knowing that I was "normal" and following a not-unusual pattern would have helped tremendously.

One month after the weaning of my third child, I began experiencing a new set of physical ailments that were totally foreign to me. I have always been blessed with good health and until the miscarriages had never undergone anything more traumatizing than removal of some wisdom teeth. Consequently, I was both surprised and concerned when I developed some rather severe bone and joint pain, which would last for days, go away, and then return. Additionally, my arms would sometimes feel as if they were numb or "asleep," and I occasionally had a great deal of pain in my lower back, pelvis, and shoulder area. As the months rolled by, the symptoms did not go away as I had thought they might. In fact, I can remember nights when I would wake up in such pain that it was necessary to take a large dosage of aspirin before I could go back to sleep. In addition to the physical symptoms I was experiencing during these times, I also felt extreme anxiety, which was undoubtedly heightened because of my puzzlement and concern over this newfound "illness."

These on-again off-again problems went on for months. When the symptoms went away (pain, anxiety, everything), I would forget that they had seemed such significant and bothersome events. It was almost like having amnesia. During the good times, I really couldn't remember that I had been so miserable. By the fourth round of symptoms, I felt that I must seek medical counsel. I started with my husband, who is a residency-trained family physician. He mentioned several possibilities, which led to some preliminary bloodwork in an effort to rule out certain diseases, including arthritis, cancer, lupus, and others. In short, all was in order in those areas. Then my husband suggested that this might be a generalized swelling problem related to my menstrual cycle. I thought he was crazy—how could my monthly period cause my arms and joints to hurt so badly that it was almost incapacitating at times? In further pursuit of answers, I had a complete neurological work-up and a "magnetic resonance imaging" study (MRI) to rule out multiple sclerosis and tumors. It was a great relief to see those tests come back negative. Because of my compounded anxiety (PMS anxiety plus fear of an unknown disease), I had become convinced that whatever I had was very bad news. With some emotional relief due to the diagnosing of what my disease "was not," I relaxed about the whole thing for a while and followed up on some reading about PMS that I had wanted to do. I was amazed to find that PMS was, in fact, much more than a monthly bout of grouchiness and water retention. There are more than a hundred symptoms that have been attributed to PMS under certain conditions. As I read about PMS in Dr. McIlhaney's first book (*1250 Health-Care Questions Women Ask* [1985]) and a few other related reference books, I became aware that every disturbing symptom I had ever had fits into this syndrome. Upon consultation with my own gynecologist, I learned that he concurred: he has patients who exhibit monthly flu-like symptoms and then recover as soon as their period starts. I felt relieved—I was getting some answers!

At this point I want to stress that not all doctors believe that PMS exists. And even some of those who acknowledge PMS do not know how to diagnose it, much less treat it. I am sure that some of the physicians I had talked to about my problem thought that I was a high-strung mother of three who just got in over her head with the birth of that third child. You know—a good case of "Shack Fever," as I have heard a mother's trials at home with small children irreverently labeled. Despite some of the negative feedback I got from a few physicians who implied that this was "all in my head," I was convinced that I was not imagining these things. They were true aches and pains—and there was a real increase in anxiety that wasn't characteristic of me, not the "normal me," anyway. This became crystal-clear to me one beautiful springtime morning when I awoke without a care and suddenly felt pain in my lower legs and arms. This was real and I was sure of it. Those pains were not figments of my imagination brought on by a fast-paced life or other external stress factors. My body was physically sick. I resolved at that moment to find out more about PMS and do whatever was possible to facilitate treatment.

I believe in taking care of the body with which I am blessed, though I certainly don't mean to suggest that mine is perfect. In my genes are tendencies toward high blood pressure, early heart disease, hypercholesterolemia, obesity, and apparently PMS. Consequently, I began my own PMS treatment program by improving my exercise and eating habits. I started a program identical to the one presented in this book for diet and exercise and experienced encouraging results almost immediately. My weight loss was gradual, not frantic. The standing joke I used on my husband was "If you had had seven pregnancies in five years, you'd need a diet, too." I now run approximately twelve miles per week and try to throw in toning exercises as time permits. Our entire family (kids included) has continued on the lo-fat, hi-fiber diet I established for myself, and we are enjoying every mouthful.

My PMS symptomology has gradually decreased over the last year from what I once considered to be almost out of control to a very tolerable and livable level of inconvenience. When premenstrual, I still lose my temper a little too much with the children, but now I am very much in control. Fatigue is absolutely nonexistent now. In fact, I can't remember a time in my entire life that I have had more energy to burn. I think the diet/exercise program can take credit for this change in my total body energy. Though we still try to plan vacations or demanding social engagements around my monthly calendar, I do not feel that my premenstrual time of the month is totally off limits. There are usually five or six days each month during which I find it necessary to take a diuretic and aspirin or ibuprofen during the height of the premenstrual phase, but I have not found it necessary to get involved with hormonal therapy at present. If my PMS were to worsen in the future, I would certainly be open to this mode of treatment.

How do I feel about PMS personally? I know it's real—I know it's physiological—I know it's a special trial for the many women who don't even know what they are struggling against. It's also hard to admit that just because I am a woman I have an inborn problem that may make me less efficient and agreeable a few days out of every month. But, unlike the avowed feminists who refuse to admit PMS exists, or those too embarrassed to even discuss this issue, I refuse to ignore it. By facing up to PMS, by accepting it as a problem that won't go away by itself, and by following the treatment plan, the "problem" has now become unimportant for me.

2

Case Studies of Women with PMS

Premenstrual syndrome can create a powerful sense of isolation. How many times have you felt alone—cut off—dissociated from friends, family, and the world around you simply because of the emotional and physical effects of monthly PMS? And, just as often, that aloneness can include a sense of separation from God. PMS can create all of these feelings. There is no denying the frustration that comes from being mentally isolated from those you love, especially when you must deal with their inability to relate to the problems you are experiencing.

Proper diagnosis and treatment must certainly be the number-one comfort factor for PMS victims. Beyond that, it can be extremely consoling simply to know that you are not alone in your trials. In fact, it is estimated that as many as 90 percent of the menstruating female population has some sort of premenstrual tension (Johnson 1987, 370). And, of that 90 percent, as many as 20 to 30 percent have *serious* problems with PMS. So, you see, if you have any premenstrual symptoms at all, you are really in the vast majority, not the minority.

Defining PMS

What exactly is premenstrual syndrome? A definition of PMS that is very simple and easily understood is "a wide variety of regularly recurring physical and psychological symptoms which occur at the same time in the premenstrual period of each cycle." This is the definition that has been proposed by Katharina Dalton (Dalton 1984), a physician in Great Britain who has had years of experience in the research and treatment of PMS. An equally important part of the PMS definition is that a woman must have one symptom-free week after menstruation is over for each monthly cycle. If her symptoms continue without that symptom-free week, her problem is not PMS but some other physical or emotional disorder.

Both of us have seen numerous patients through the years who fit this general description of PMS. However, since PMS is a "syndrome," every patient's case is different. A syndrome is a clinical term for a problem that is really a collection of many symptoms—of which you may personally have a few or many. Some women's symptoms may be mild, while others' are severe. Your own struggles with PMS may vary greatly from those of a neighbor or friend.

The term *premenstrual syndrome* applies to those women who are having menstrual periods. However, women who have had a hysterectomy but still have their ovaries can have premenstrual-type symptoms, even though they no longer menstruate. This is because their ovaries are still producing the normal female hormonal cycle that can cause them to have feelings associated with PMS.

Christian Women with PMS

Although the information and treatment program presented in this book can be applied to all women, we particularly want to help Christian women with PMS, since this condition seems to foster many spiritual dilemmas. Christian women are often confused about the possible relationship between their spiritual life and the presence of premenstrual tension. If you feel the comfort of the Holy Spirit during the good times of the month, you may wonder where that comfort is when you are at your wit's end and close to losing control during your premenstrual days. The answer is that the Spirit is still with you, but your body feels so bad that it is difficult to feel God's comfort. Many PMS women may have feelings of great anger or despair. Others feel quite ill, as if they had flu symptoms every fourth week. Some feel pushed to the outer edge of tolerance and control, while others are only mildly inconvenienced. Whatever the case may be, we would like to point out right now that *PMS is not a spiritual problem.* Whether or not a woman is in fellowship with God, she may experience symptoms of PMS so disturbing that she feels "unspiritual" at the time. The fact is, she can still be in fellowship with God though her general feeling is one of discomfort, unrest, disharmony, and anger. Our attempt in pointing this out is to take away any unnecessary concern about your faith system. Don't let needless guilt over your lack of spirituality be an additional burden to carry as you deal with the physical problems of PMS. Remember that the vast majority of menstruating women, whether Christian or not, may be affected by PMS to some extent. You are definitely not an isolated statistic. And God has promised not to leave you "comfortless."

Potential Consequences of Untreated PMS

This growing nationwide concern over PMS is not academic. PMS can cause havoc within your personal relationships and is possibly dangerous for your overall health. A study by Drs. MacKinnon, MacKinnon, and Thomson reported in 1959 on a hundred consecutive women dying of suicide, accidental death, and natural causes. It was noted that 89 percent of the suicides and 90 percent of the accident victims died during the two weeks prior to their menstrual period—the PMS time. Perhaps more surprisingly, 64 percent of the women dying of natural causes also died during their premenstrual days. Certainly more information on this significant correlation is needed. However, it is an indication that getting control over your PMS may be a life-or-death matter, besides being of vital importance to your emotional and physical well-being, your productivity, and your relationships with the significant people in your life.

Patients with PMS

The previous brief overview of PMS should serve as an orientation to the problem, but we also feel that you can benefit from reading about the experiences of other women with PMS. It is important for you to note, as you read through the following actual patient stories, that we discussed many forms of treatment with these women. We did not just prescribe drugs. We spent time with these women, encouraging dietary modification and emphasizing the importance of a regular exercise program. We also talked about how to live with their own cycles, not against them. Essentially, we educated these patients in the various treatments we will later discuss in greater detail. Conquering PMS involves careful attention to all the facets of treatment that make up a complete PMS program.

Obviously, just as the severity and type of symptoms vary in any physiologically based syndrome, so does the plan of treatment. What works with one woman who has PMS may not work with another. Although we will discuss many self-help measures, it should be understood that the starting point should be a complete physical work-up supervised by a trusted and sympathetic physician. You may, indeed, have PMS—but it is important to rule out other causative factors and tailor your treatment to your overall physical condition and lifestyle.

Patient One: "I even called the suicide hotline"

This married woman (31) has never had children. She has had a tubal ligation for sterilization purposes. She vividly described her symptoms:

> I turn into a basket case starting one week prior to my period, and this lasts through the week of my period. I am rotten and mean like a snake. Even now, when I'm talking about it, it is like I am talking about someone else. It is horrible. It is awful. Last month was the worst. I could think of no reason to live and even called the suicide hotline. I have no interest in sex, and my husband blames this on the tubal ligation. I have no patience at all and really can't believe the things that I hear myself saying. One day I'll be fine and then it's like a wave rolling over me. Once I just sat on the floor in the kitchen for about an hour and a half and didn't even know I had been there.
>
> When the PMS is over I can never decide if I need to go to the doctor or not, because then I feel fine. For the rest of the month I'll be okay; then it starts all over again.
>
> When I took birth-control pills (prior to tubal ligation) I felt really bad. I noticed that on the thirteenth day of each cycle I was paranoid, depressed, mean, and crazy. Sometimes I felt like I was losing my equilibrium.

Treatment. This patient was initially treated with Efamol and progesterone suppositories. This helped somewhat. With the later addition of Xanex (an anti-anxiety agent), she noted further improvement in her symptoms.

Patient Two: "I yell a lot"

Here was a woman (35) with two children. Her husband called before her first visit to explain that his wife was so "horrible" during the days before her period that this was causing significant marital problems. When she came to my office, she had the following words to say:

> I yell a lot the week before my period and hardly ever get upset at any other time. Once I actually picked up the television and threw it at my husband I was so angry.

Treatment. This patient was treated with a combination of medications, including vitamin B_6, progesterone suppositories, spironolactone, and Ponstel. The treatment was complicated by the fact that initially the patient would call the office during her premenstrual time and say that she was very upset and couldn't really remember or understand how she was to take her medication. Carefully written instructions and the help of a concerned family member helped improve this patient's compliance with the prescribed treatment.

Patient Three: "I feel like my body is swollen"

This woman (32) had three children and had this to say:

> Since my last child was born one year ago I've had a lot of pain on my right side from the time of ovulation until my period starts. During this time I also feel very nervous and on edge. I'll cry a lot, have headaches, feel like my body is swollen, and get my feelings hurt real easy.

Treatment. The use of vitamin B_6 and Ponstel during the PMS time almost completely relieved this patient's symptoms within one month of treatment.

Patient Four: "The cramps are really bad"

A mother (34) of two children describes her PMS:

> I have severe cramping from the twelfth day of my period on. The cramps are really bad during the five or six

> days just before my period. I also feel a lot of tension, abdominal bloating, breast tenderness, lack of energy, and some nausea.

Treatment. Initial treatment of this patient included Ponstel and vitamin B_6. Good results had been obtained within one month but the symptoms of swelling persisted. The addition of spironolactone alleviated this problem.

Patient Five: "My breasts hurt"

This description from a mother (45) of four children:

> Two weeks before every period I feel moody, irritable, clumsy, forgetful, and dizzy. My breasts hurt and I feel real swollen. These symptoms have been very bad for about a year now, and the funny thing is that within a few hours of my period's start I feel just fine.

Treatment. Ponstel, Diuril (a diuretic), vitamin B_6, and Efamol were prescribed for the first six months of therapy. Unfortunately the patient's symptoms persisted, and her condition worsened to the point where she felt extremely frustrated, paranoid, and even had suicidal thoughts during her PMS time. Increasing dosages of progesterone suppositories and an exercise program were begun. We wanted to try Danocrine with this patient, but she felt it was too expensive. Instead we added Xanex, and the patient soon called back to report that it was really helping. After spironolactone was added to help with some residual swelling, the patient reported that she was doing really great, even on the day before her period.

PMS in Adolescence

It is noteworthy that Sharon has traced the beginnings of her own PMS symptoms to the teenage years. In his recent film series "Turn Your Heart Toward Home,"

Dr. James Dobson, eminent author and president of Focus on the Family, points out that much of the unrest and disharmony teenagers cause in their homes and families may be the result of hormonal changes that occur in their bodies. He adds that in females this can often include PMS. He suggests that if adolescent girls are causing a great deal of turbulence in the home, the time of those events be noted to detect any correlations with the premenstrual week. The two of us could not agree more with his comments.

3

History, Causes, and Incidence of PMS

Premenstrual syndrome could have been called the medical topic of the year in 1982, when it was widely featured on nationwide talk shows and in magazines and newspapers stories. Since then, PMS has become a popular topic at medical conferences. Is this really a disease of the Eighties, or are we just more aware today that PMS, though part of being a woman, is a treatable medical problem? One physician has stated that PMS is "the world's commonest, and probably oldest disease" (Dalton 1984, viii). Though we would not agree that PMS is actually a "disease," we agree with her statement.

History of PMS

The "oldest disease"—that is an interesting idea. Was Eve irritable on a monthly basis? The female menstrual cycle has even been referred to as "Eve's Curse," not that there is necessarily any connection. But Eve's role in the fall from grace seems to make her an easy target for blame.

Historically, there has been mystique, legend, and fear associated with the menstrual cycle. Records of ancient societies reveal that menstruation was connected with ill fortune, disasters, and the supernatural. People who did not understand the physiological function of the menstrual cycle found it absolutely fearful that a woman could bleed for several days each month and continue to thrive (Norris 1984). To them, blood meant death. Even the Greek philosopher Aristotle commented that the "glance of a menstrual woman takes the polish from a mirror and the person who glances in it will be bewitched" (Norris 1984).

The first suggestions that the menstrual period and PMS are, in fact, physiologic occurrences were made by Hippocrates (c. 460–377 B.C.), the father of modern medicine. He pointed out that women could experience troublesome physical and psychological symptoms during the days before their menstrual periods (Barber 1986). Another twenty-three centuries passed before a serious attempt was made to validate this observation. R. T. Frank, in an article called "Hormonal Causes of Premenstrual Tension," published in *The Archives of Neurologic Psychiatry,* described fifteen women with a number of different complaints related to the premenstrual time (Frank 1931). The term *PMS,* or *premenstrual syndrome,* was coined in 1953 by Dr. Katharina Dalton, a physician living in Great Britain who has since popularized the use of progesterone in PMS treatment.

With such a negative heritage associated with the monthly period, it is little wonder that it has taken so long for this subject to be discussed rationally and without embarrassment. Even the medical profession has been slow to understand the true nature and causes of PMS. L. Gannon reported in *Menstrual Disorders and Menopause* that twenty-five years after Frank's first PMS article, statements like the following were still being made:

> A consideration of the main syndromes of menstrual disturbance is inseparable from that of the question of

> the relationship between disturbance and neurosis [Gregory, 1957, 65].
>
> Many patients present gynecological symptoms without being sick. Their illness represents a psychic conflict sailing under a gynecologic flag . . . [Rogers, 1950, 322].

Fortunately for PMS victims, there has been a definite shift from considering the syndrome as a psychologically based disorder to identifying it as having an organic nature. Perhaps we should not be too hard on the doctors and researchers of the 1950s and 1960s, however. They thought that all obesity was psychological in origin, too! It is common for ideas and research to glide in one direction for many years, based on supposition alone. It seems to take many years for old theories to die and newer and more accurate ones to take their place. This is why you will still find physicians who think that PMS is "all in your head."

The entrance of greater numbers of females into the realm of medicine and scientific research may have made an impact on understanding PMS in recent years. There is no denying that a personal experience with PMS symptoms will convince a person of its organic reality.

Ironically, even some women have been skeptical about PMS. They chide other women for their inability to cope with PMS and label them "weak-willed." Radical feminists seem to want the entire issue to go away, since they see PMS as a detriment to the furtherance of women's rights and overall respect in the workplace. For many women, PMS is more of a problem of denial than misconception. They know PMS is real; they just seem to have amnesia after each period and deny that they may have a medical problem that requires treatment. We all sometimes need reminding that denial will never be an effective treatment for a medical ailment.

If you think you have PMS, accept it and start on the road to treatment now. Don't settle for as little as one good week each month, when you might be able to have three or four. Don't settle, either, for feeling okay instead of great or for just barely handling your daily responsibilities because you are limited by your premenstrual symptoms. We certainly don't have all the answers, yet; but the treatment we suggest will offer you practical ideas that will help you to conquer some of those PMS-related problems.

Causes of PMS

Most of us use the term *premenstrual syndrome* (or its abbreviation, PMS) because it plainly describes the problem. The term merely says that there is a condition that occurs before a woman's monthly period that may cause her to feel ill. The name is obviously used because we don't really know what causes PMS or what causes some women to have severe PMS while others have symptoms that are hardly noticeable.

We both believe that PMS is a "normal" condition, since it affects such a large percentage of the female population (as many as 95 percent). However, perhaps there *are* disease patterns at work in those who have the most severe symptoms. For your intellectual curiosity, we have listed some of the most predominant theories about the possible cause(s) of PMS:

1. Progesterone deficiency
2. Estrogen deficiency
3. Abnormalities of the estrogen/progesterone ratio
4. Subclinical thyroid deficiency
5. Increased progesterone-type androgens (Some of the male-type hormones in a woman's body originate from progesterone compounds in her body.)
6. Decreased levels of vitamin B_6 in the body
7. Decreased levels of vitamin A in the body

8. Decreased levels of vitamin E in the body
9. Decreased levels of magnesium in the body
10. Abnormal essential fatty acid metabolism
11. Altered carbohydrate tolerance
12. Elevated aldosterone levels
13. Endogenous opiate withdrawal (All people have opiate-like hormones present in their bodies, and it seems that some women are sensitive to the body's withdrawing the normal level of these opiates and that the decreased levels that are present premenstrually cause a woman's body to feel ill.)
14. Progesterone allergy
15. Neuro-transmitter abnormalities (Ovarian hormones and neuro-transmitters are both responsible for regulating sexual behavior and ovulation. It may be that neuro-transmitters are not working properly in women who have severe PMS. Studies in this area have hardly even begun but will include evaluation of monoamines, which include serotonin and dopamine, and also studies of acetylcholine.)
16. Generalized yeast infection (In the book *The Yeast Connection* [Crook 1985], a whole body yeast infection was touted as the cause for PMS and many other ailments. We do not feel that this is a likely cause of PMS and have not seen this to be true among our own patients. We mention it only to inform you.)

This list of possible causes of PMS may mean very little to you. It actually means very little to most physicians involved in treating PMS as well. Until the true causes are known, the important aspects of PMS will be very personal and practical: get it diagnosed and treated.

Incidence of PMS

For most women with PMS, it is somehow a relief to know that as many as 95 percent of all women are affected to some degree by premenstrual symptoms. It seems unlikely to us that God would have designed a woman's body so that this large a percentage of women would have a hormonal disease! Many researchers now believe that PMS is not a disease at all, but a normal reaction of a woman's body to the hormonal changes that are going on inside of her.

Perhaps we can find an analogy in adolescent acne. We can accept acne as a not-uncommon occurrence during adolescence. We also realize that some adolescents have more trouble than others, just as some women have more severe cases of PMS. In spite of the fact that we consider teenage acne "normal," we still go to physicians for treatment so that the emotional and physical scarring that can result from acne may be lessened. In the same way, the less-severe cases of PMS should be understood by women as a normal process, though not necessarily a desired one. The most severe cases may actually be some sort of hormonal disease, but no one knows that yet. Thankfully, both the mild and severe forms of PMS respond to treatment.

Even though PMS may be a non-pathological component of a woman's being, it can produce severe problems in some individuals. One estimate is that as many as 30 percent of all menstruating women are actually "incapacitated" by their PMS during the days before their period starts. That's three out of every ten women you meet! We certainly don't have all the answers as to why PMS affects almost all women to some degree. We do, however, feel that diet, exercise, certain medical treatments—and prayer—can help women deal with it more positively.

The following information is provided to complete your knowledge about the incidence of PMS and its relationship to age and hereditary factors.

Age Factors

The Teenage Years. Many practitioners believe that the symptoms of PMS frequently start during puberty. Somehow it seems easy to neglect this tumultuous group who have just given up their toys for more "grown-up" activities. Estimates of the incidence of the syndrome in adolescents vary from 20–30 percent of the teenagers who visit physicians (Norris 1984, 164). On the other hand, this figure might actually be much higher, since many teenagers are either too embarrassed to discuss menstrual problems or are unaware that their newly experienced monthly period could be related to their recurrent fatigue and irritability. In short, most of them just don't want to talk about it! Physicians are just now becoming aware that PMS problems may have their inception at these early ages. In Ronald Norris's book *Premenstrual Syndrome* (1984), he states of another physician: "One pediatrician in Boston, a patient of ours, says she has observed a great number of girls with PMS in her practice; since she's undergone the evaluation process herself she's been able to diagnose them and refer them for treatment."

Though parents rarely consider the possibility of PMS in their adolescent daughters, the documentation of irritable and rebellious behavior on a cyclic, monthly basis might be convincing evidence. Then, by simply counseling the teen on some of the treatment measures we suggest, the problem may improve. A parent should take care not to use PMS as the scapegoat for all poor behavior, however. No one wants to encourage a teenage girl or anyone else to avoid responsibilities with an attitude of "I can't help it—I have PMS."

The Twenties and Thirties. PMS may increase slightly in the twenties but seems to increase markedly by the thirties (Dalton 1984). Reasons for this occurrence are unclear, but it seems probable that it results from a combination of internal factors (perhaps hormonal changes) and the added external stress that may accompany these particular years of life. Whether one is a full-time mother and homemaker, is on a fast-track career ladder, or is trying to juggle the two roles, women of the eighties must deal with more stress than ever before. The media never lets you be anything less than perfect, even when dealing with preschoolers, a demanding job, and the "Battle of the Bulge." What a burden!

Most Christian women especially desire not to "give in" to lifestyle pressures brought on by a self-oriented world. We all hope that we can keep our thoughts and eyes on Christ. The fact is, though, that most of us will feel stress from these worldly pressures from time to time. The connection with PMS is that added stress seems to heighten PMS symptoms, especially those related to tension. Anxiety can mount to such heights as to create or contribute to situations causing marital problems, divorce, child abuse, alcoholism, and other external evidence of unhappy lives.

Additionally, some clinicians (Norris 1984) feel that having pregnancies and miscarriages, as well as using birth-control pills, may contribute toward PMS symptoms. Thus, since these times of hormonal change usually occur during the twenties and thirties, PMS is more common or pronounced in these two decades.

The Forties. Though the byword of many clinicians (and the hope of many women in their thirties) is that PMS improves in the forties, there is no conclusive evidence to support this supposition. To quote one authority (Norris 1984, 177): "For most women with premenstrual syndrome, even untreated, the forties is usually the beginning of the end. The worst is over in terms of severity and duration of symptoms, and for most women PMS will end with menopause." However, directly before this quote, the author cites a case study of a forty-four-year-old woman whose life dramatically changed for the better when treated for premenstrual syndrome.

During the past few years, the observation of women in their late thirties or in their forties seems to indicate that women have an increasing chance of having PMS or having their symptoms worsen right up until menopause. Recent unpublished studies suggest that PMS is actually due to inadequate estrogen levels in a woman's body. Since these later years of a woman's reproductive life (about age 40 on) are associated with gradually decreasing estrogen levels, perhaps worsening PMS should be expected with increasing age.

In a study by Dr. Olaf Widholm, a professor in the department of obstetrics and gynecology at the Central Hospital of Helsinki University in Finland (Kantero and Widholm 1971), over five thousand adolescent girls and their mothers (age thirty-five to forty-five) were studied by means of a questionnaire that concerned menstrual patterns. He states: "The combination of dysmenorrhea and premenstrual tension was reported by 62 percent of the mothers. This apparently constitutes a considerable stress on middle-age women."

The Menopausal Years. There is very little clear-cut information concerning the relationship of premenstrual syndrome and the menopausal woman. As is the case in much of the available PMS literature, the current research is based on individual case studies rather than large numbers of patients in a closely supervised situation. Some clinicians feel that PMS decreases during the forties and certainly the fifties. Others, however, feel that the opposite is true.

Distinction between menopausal symptoms and PMS is usually clear. The usual menopausal complaints—hot flashes, vaginal dryness, and the like—are not cyclical. However, some menopausal women may suffer simultaneous PMS symptoms (Norris 1984). There may even be a few women whose PMS seems to begin at menopause. In such cases, it usually becomes evident that these women had mild PMS prior to menopause but did not recognize it at the time. The PMS symptoms most frequently seen at this age include irritability, vague muscle and joint aches, fatigue, and lack of concentration, but they may include any of the symptoms listed elsewhere in his book.

We are using the term *menopause* here the way most nonmedical people use it, meaning the period of time during which a woman's ovaries are failing and continuing until there are no more periods. Technically, this is the first half of a woman's climacteric and the term *menopause* actually means a woman's last period. Used in this technical sense, after a woman's menopause, she could no longer have premenstrual syndrome because her ovaries have essentially become "dead" and are almost totally inactive.

Hereditary Factors

There is apparently a genetically determined factor involved in PMS. Dalton (1984) reports that sixteen pairs of female twins were evaluated for premenstrual syndrome. Their diagnoses were made by menstrual charts, and all were affected severely enough to require medical treatment. Six of the seven pairs of *identical* twins exhibited PMS in both sisters, whereas in only three of the nine sets of *nonidentical* twins did both sisters have PMS. As Dalton points out, although the small sample size of this study is not statistically significant, it is suggestive of a genetic factor.

As previously noted, Kantero and Widholm (1971) studied premenstrual symptomology in adolescent daughters and their mothers. They noted that 63 percent of the daughters of symptom-free mothers were also symptom-free. On the other hand, if the mothers had premenstrual fatigue or irritability, nearly 70 percent of the daughters had similar symptoms. Furthermore:

> The comparison of the mother/daughter menstrual patterns indicated that the symptoms of pain, or the lack of them were obviously repeated from mother to daughter. Both genetic factors and unconscious imitation may play an important part in the etiology of both dysmenorrhea and premenstrual tension. The correlation coefficient of menstrual patterns between daughters and their mothers was highly significant, a finding which to some extent speaks in favor of a genetic influence.

Dalton (1984, 96) has also noted that adopted daughters tend to have the same type of menstrual cycle as their natural mothers rather than their adoptive mothers, indicating that this is not a learned pattern, but a response to physiological similarities.

In the final analysis, you must be wondering if you will suffer from premenstrual syndrome because your mother did. Our best estimate, based on current data, is that you will have a 60 to 70 percent chance of following in your mother's footsteps in that respect. That is, if she had painful menstruation and premenstrual tension, more than likely so will you. Further, if your mother has had symptom-free periods, then so may you.

Part 2

Diagnosing PMS

4

Identifying Your Symptoms

As we have noted, premenstrual syndrome has only recently been accepted within the medical community as a bona fide physical problem. You may find this hard to believe, especially if you suffer from PMS. How could medical science not have realized the reality of PMS sooner? Part of the reason for this situation may be because opinions have varied greatly as to what PMS actually includes. Most physicians would now agree that there is a problem called PMS and that a good definition for it has been written by Dr. K. Dalton: "a wide variety of regularly recurring physical and psychological symptoms which occur at the same time in the premenstrual period of each cycle."

Not only does this definition provide agreement for medical personnel concerning PMS, but it also helps people suffering from PMS understand what it is. To fully understand this definition, however, we must first understand both the basics of the female menstrual cycle and the symptoms classified as PMS. Both of these basics will be discussed in this chapter.

The Female Cycle

A woman's monthly cycle is one of the most fascinating and delicately balanced systems of the human female body.

Though there are some uncomfortable side effects such as PMS, monthly passage of blood, and so on, still the reproductive cycle is a marvel of God's creation.

There is a more exhaustive review of the woman's menstrual cycle in chapter 5. For now we will begin by saying that the cycle normally lasts twenty-eight days. Doctors usually consider the woman's cycle as beginning with "Day 1," the first day of her menstrual flow, which typically lasts five days. Fourteen days after the blood flow starts, ovulation normally occurs (this is "Day 14" of the cycle).

At ovulation, the woman's ovaries begin producing progesterone, and this may be one of the causes for PMS. In some yet-unknown way, the production of progesterone may be associated with the onset of premenstrual symptoms, which means that PMS can continue from the time of ovulation until the onset of the period (the next "Day 1"). Some women do not experience symptoms until a day or two before their period starts. Other women have PMS for the entire two weeks prior to the onset of their period. Still others experience a peak of symptoms right after ovulation, followed by milder symptoms for the remaining ten to twelve days. Most women stop having symptoms of PMS as soon as their period starts; but some continue to have PMS for two or three days into the period or even until the blood flow stops. After the cessation of menstrual bleeding, PMS symptoms completely disappear until ovulation occurs, usually seven to nine days later. These symptom-free days are essential for the diagnosis of PMS. *If a woman does not experience these good days, she probably does not have PMS.*

Symptoms of PMS

"How would I feel if I had PMS?" In other words, "What are the symptoms of PMS?" That is indeed a difficult question, since it is not entirely known to what extent and in what manner PMS affects different women. In the tables below, we have provided an exhaustive list of the PMS symptoms both reported by other researchers and seen in our own practices. Some of these symptoms affect almost all women at some time, while others may be rare, even among PMS patients. Also, since so little is known about the syndrome, and the specific cause is undiscovered, the symptom lists are probably incomplete. You may find yourself described in this list. One word of caution: *Don't let PMS become a catch-all diagnosis for your ailments.* The key is that your symptoms must disappear completely for at least one week following your menstrual period. Otherwise, it is *not* PMS, and you should seek medical help for treatment of some other condition that may or may not be serious.

As you check the list below, mark the symptoms you most often experience during the premenstrual days. We will use this information in the next section. Identifying your symptoms will help you to know what to do about them when treatments are discussed.

Physical Symptoms

- ☐ abdominal bloating
- ☐ fullness in the lower abdomen
- ☐ aching in the lower abdomen
- ☐ generalized swelling of the body
- ☐ tightness of rings
- ☐ tightness of shoes
- ☐ tingling in the fingers (parasthesias)
- ☐ carpal tunnel syndrome (numbness of the hands related to swelling in the wrists)
- ☐ breast tenderness
- ☐ headaches
- ☐ acne

- [ ] skin rashes
- [ ] irritation of the eyes (conjunctivitis)
- [ ] irritation of the eyes not caused by infection
- [ ] outbreaks of herpes (including fever blisters of the lips or herpes of the vulvar area)
- [ ] sinus congestion (due to increased fluid production from the sinuses)
- [ ] increased vaginal secretions (a woman may think she has a vaginal infection)
- [ ] increased problems with pre-existent epilepsy
- [ ] increased problems with asthma (not a cause, but symptoms may worsen)
- [ ] backache
- [ ] muscle-spasms and pain in the arms and legs, especially the joints
- [ ] passing-out episodes (syncope)
- [ ] tiredness and fatigue
- [ ] dizziness
- [ ] lack of coordination
- [ ] clumsiness
- [ ] heart palpitations
- [ ] poorly-fitting dentures
- [ ] easy bruising
- [ ] increased problems with hypoglycemia or with feelings of hypoglycemia
- [ ] increased problems with ulcerative colitis
- [ ] increased problems with pre-existent heart disease
- [ ] ulcerations of the mouth

Emotional Symptoms

- [ ] tension
- [ ] irritability

- [ ] depression
- [ ] anxiety
- [ ] mood swings
- [ ] outbursts of temper
- [ ] shouting
- [ ] throwing things
- [ ] paranoia
- [ ] forgetfulness
- [ ] self-blaming
- [ ] desire to withdraw from other people
- [ ] suicidal feeling
- [ ] compulsive activity
- [ ] change in sexual interest (usually increased at the time of ovulation and decreased afterward)
- [ ] aggression
- [ ] lethargy
- [ ] sleeping disorders
- [ ] insomnia
- [ ] nightmares or unusual dreams
- [ ] unnatural fears
- [ ] increased use of alcohol and other mood-altering drugs
- [ ] argumentativeness
- [ ] inability to initiate activities or accomplish work at the usual pace
- [ ] indecisiveness (or the making of poor decisions)
- [ ] marital conflict
- [ ] food cravings
- [ ] increased appetite
- [ ] difficulty in concentrating

Timing Is the Key. You probably noticed that we separated PMS symptoms into two groups. This is our own classification, but to us it seems reasonable and helpful. The separation is not a totally scientific one, however. For instance, it may be that a difficulty in concentration is not an emotional problem but a physical response caused by the swelling of brain tissue during the PMS days. The important thing in attributing any of these symptoms to PMS is that they occur before (and possibly during) the menstrual period, and that you be absolutely free of them as soon as your menstrual period is over. Additionally, these symptoms will not return until after the time of ovulation. Thus, PMS symptoms occur only during the fourteen days before the period and perhaps during the first few days of the menstrual bleeding. If these symptoms occur at any other time, they are not due to PMS but to some other problem.

Different Symptoms for Different Women. Again, the amount of difficulty that women have with PMS varies greatly. Some may be totally incapacitated with each monthly cycle. Other women may only have one symptom, which only mildly bothers them. There is great variation in both the number of symptoms a woman may have and in how much they bother her. In the clinic we have seen patients with a list of twenty PMS symptoms, all of which are very bothersome. Alternatively, we have seen women who are discomforted merely by the fact that they experience swelling for three or four days before their menstrual period. If your own personal symptoms are weighing heavily upon your mind, do something about it! Start by reading all the chapters in this book and implementing changes that pertain to you. (It is wise to consult your physician first, especially if you have another medical problem.) Don't be content to suffer during one, two, or three weeks out of every month for the rest of your menstruating life. Seek solutions. If these changes do not make a difference, seek your physician's advice again.

Finding Out from Someone Else. Ironically, you may be the only person in your family or working circle who fails to recognize your PMS problem. When someone tries to tell you that they think you have PMS, you may feel offended and hurt. That is a completely understandable reaction. None of us likes to hear anything negative about ourselves. Try to remember that this is not criticism. Be willing to listen to those around you, including your friends, the people with whom you work, and certainly your children or your husband. Are they asking you why you seem "grouchy" at certain times each month? If these symptoms are interfering with important relationships in your life, you need evaluation and treatment. This is a very important point, since many PMS specialists attribute a higher incidence of divorce, separation, and child abuse to women suffering from PMS. It is also important that those people who do the "pointing out" of your problems do so in a loving manner and during the time of your cycle when PMS is not present. You will then be calmer and more receptive to what they are telling you. If they point out your symptoms during your troublesome premenstrual phase, you may be literally incapable of accepting the fact that the way you are feeling is due to PMS. During that time of the month, you will often be absolutely certain that the way you feel is the result of unfair attitudes from those around you, or your unsatisfying situation in life.

Common Threads

There are some physical characteristics that women with PMS may have in common. Though this information is presented in several popular references (Norris 1984, 10–11; Harrison 1985, 12), it is not generally found in the professional research articles. Many physicians who treat PMS have noticed that chronic PMS sufferers may share some common experiences and characteristics:

Usually pain-free menstruation

Symptoms beginning at puberty, after pregnancy, at onset or termination of birth-control pills, or in association with other major hormonal events

Increased severity of PMS after pregnancy or after cessation of breastfeeding

Absence of PMS symptoms during last six months of pregnancy

Pregnancy complications, including miscarriage, toxemia, and postpartum depression

Symptoms may leave abruptly with the start of the menstrual period

Symptoms may be more or less severe on different months

Symptoms worsen with age

Inability to tolerate the birth-control pill

Intolerance for alcohol premenstrually

Food cravings and premenstrual overeating

Monthly weight fluctuations

A history of female family members with similar PMS problems

Charting Your Symptoms

You may ask, "How can I know if I am suffering from PMS? Do I have to wait for my friends and family to tell me about it?" If you suspect that you might have PMS, there is a simple step you can take to confirm or deny your suspicions. Then your doctor can either validate your suspicions or determine that you are suffering from some other ailment that causes similar complaints.

The most reliable method of diagnosing PMS is to chart your symptoms on a PMS calendar, such as the one provided in this chapter. We have already stressed that timing is key. To prove the cyclic nature of your symptoms, you must be prepared to keep a careful and objective record of their occurrence for at least three months. If you can do this prior to seeing a physician, that may save you time and money. In fact, accurate charting of your PMS symptoms is the most important step you can personally take to get proper diagnosis. Remember, if your symptoms are not consistently occurring at the pertinent time within your monthly cycle, you don't have PMS.

Instructions for Using the PMS Calendar

1. If possible, make a few photocopies of the PMS calendar before beginning, so you can recheck your cycles in six or more months.
2. Look at the list of physical and emotional symptoms given earlier in this chapter. Check or highlight the five symptoms that seem to consistently give you the most difficulty. Then use a code for recording those symptoms, such as "T" for tension or "BT" for breast tenderness.
3. Begin recording these codes on your PMS calendar at the end of your next menstrual period. Always record your symptoms on the day they occur. Don't try to remember how you felt several days before or make a single recording at the end of the week. Also, if the symptoms are mild to moderate, write them in small letters; if they worsen or are severe, record them in capital letters.
4. Mark your menstrual flow days with a circled "M."
5. Keep this record for three consecutive menstrual cycles.

Evaluation of Your PMS Calendar

Now let's look at the PMS calendar examples. If your calendar begins to look like Chart "A" in the PMS calendar—where most of the symptoms are grouped in the fourteen days preceeding the menstrual flow—you probably do have PMS. Note that although Chart "A" represents only one cycle, you should keep your calendar for *three* cycles to get the best diagnosis. On the other hand,

A PMS Calendar

Use this type of calendar to record your *five worst symptoms.* Two sample months are shown at right.

Examples of coding

A—Anxiety

AB—Abdominal Bloating

BT—Breast Tenderness

H—Headache

M—Menstruation

	Month 1	Month 2	Month 3
1			
2			
3			
4			
5			
6			
7			
8			
9			
10			
11			
12			
13			
14			
15			
16			
17			
18			
19			
20			
21			
22			
23			
24			
25			
26			
27			
28			
29			
30			
31			
32			
33			
34			
35			

In Chart "A" the woman is diagnosed as having PMS. In Chart "B" the timing of symptoms does not have a clear relationship to the menstrual cycle; this woman's symptoms may have another cause that should be investigated.

	Chart A	Chart B
1		
2		a
3	h	A
4		
5		a
6		
7		
8		H
9		
10		
11		
12		
13		
14	A	
15	HA 6+	H
16	a	a
17	a	
18	A	A
19	Ah	
20	Ha AB	
21	HAB	
22	HAB (M)	(H)
23	AB (M)	
24	(M)	(M)
25	(M)	(M)
26	(M)	(M)
27		(M)
28		(M)
29		h
30		
31	H	A
32		
33		
34		
35		

if your symptoms are scattered throughout the month, as the example of Chart "B" shows, your problems are probably related to something other than PMS.

If you decide to see a doctor about your PMS, take this chart with you. It will be of real help in diagnosing your symptoms.

5

The Menstrual Cycle—A Physiological Review

Hold on to your thinking caps, because we're going to take you through a whirlwind review of female physiology. Even though this chapter is scientifically oriented and may seem less than practical, most women feel a great need to understand exactly what happens to their bodies each month. What are the hormones that are causing these changes? What is ovulation? How do you know when you are premenstrual? These questions and many more will be answered in this chapter.

Overview of the Female Menstrual Cycle

The normal menstrual period lasts for five days. In general, fourteen days after a woman starts her menstrual period, she ovulates (releases an egg from one of her ovaries). After another fourteen days, she will start her period again, and the cycle goes on through her childbearing years. Remember, some women's menstrual cycles will be much more irregular than this. Some women will bleed for only two days and others for seven days or longer. It is also fairly common for a woman's menstrual periods to come every thirty to thirty-five days, or for menstruation to be somewhat "irregular."

A girl's ovaries begin producing estrogens several months before she starts having menstrual periods. This is why her breasts usually develop before menstrual periods begin. The estrogen comes from small fluid-filled sacs in the ovaries called *follicles*. At *menarche* (the time when a woman begins her menstrual periods), the ovaries collectively contain over 300,000 immature eggs. Then with each period during the reproductive age of life, the body takes fourteen days to mature one of those eggs for expulsion from the ovary. This process is called *ovulation*.

The follicle from which the egg is released then becomes the *corpus luteum*, a cystic structure that secretes both estrogen and progesterone. It is at this phase—after ovulation and when progesterone secretion is elevated—that a woman can develop PMS. In some yet-undetermined way, PMS seems somehow related to the presence of progesterone in a woman's body. Significant amounts of progesterone are not present until ovulation occurs. Fourteen days later, if a woman does not become pregnant, she begins her menstrual period because the corpus luteum has become "old" in only fourteen days and can no longer produce adequate amounts of estrogen and progesterone to keep the woman from sloughing off the uterine lining (which had been prepared for the reception of a fertilized egg). As these hormone levels drop precipitously, the woman starts her menstrual periods all over again. The graph below shows the hormonal changes we have just discussed.

We have already mentioned that some women have cycles that do not span exactly twenty-eight days. In fact, menstrual cycles may range from only twenty days to as long as thirty-five days and still be considered normal. The important thing to remember is that ovulation occurs fourteen days *before* the menstrual period starts, regardless of the total length of the cycle. For example, if a

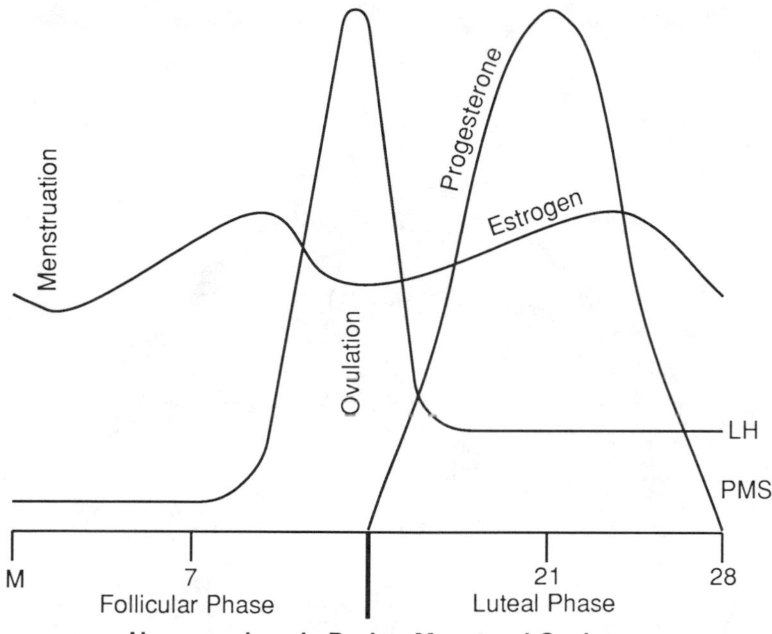

Hormone Levels During Menstrual Cycle

woman has a period every thirty-five days, she ovulates fourteen days before the thirty-fifth day of her cycle. Remember, we always count the days of the menstrual cycle from the day the period starts. As mentioned in chapter 4, that first day of menstrual bleeding is Day 1. A woman with a regular thirty-five-day cycle who is ovulating normally would not have any PMS symptoms until Day 21 of her cycle and thereafter (until her period starts). If she has symptoms at any other time during the month, they are not PMS-related and cannot be successfully treated as PMS. The chart on the next page depicts the physiological changes for a cycle of twenty-eight days.

The Four Phases of the Menstrual Cycle

The following diagram depicts the various phases in a normal menstrual cycle. These phases will be explained further in the rest of the chapter.

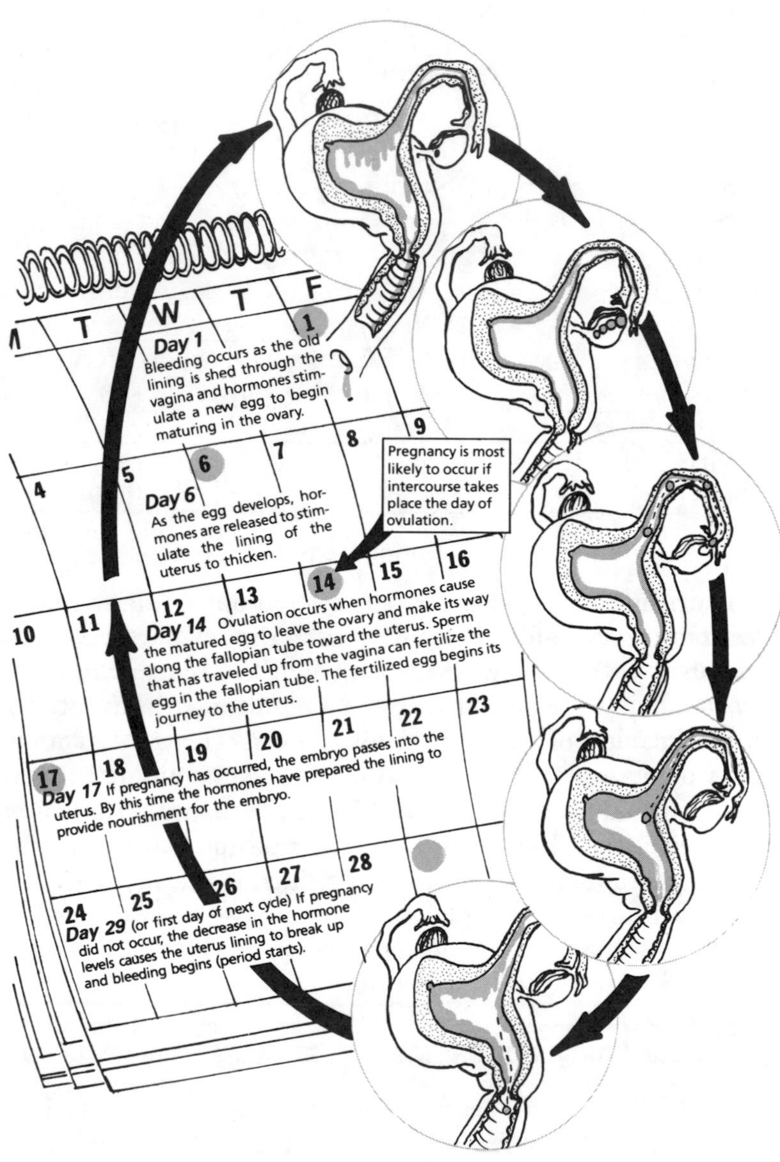
M T W T F
1
Day 1 Bleeding occurs as the old lining is shed through the vagina and hormones stimulate a new egg to begin maturing in the ovary.
4 5 6 7 8 9
Day 6 As the egg develops, hormones are released to stimulate the lining of the uterus to thicken.
Pregnancy is most likely to occur if intercourse takes place the day of ovulation.
10 11 12 13 14 15 16
Day 14 Ovulation occurs when hormones cause the matured egg to leave the ovary and make its way along the fallopian tube toward the uterus. Sperm that has traveled up from the vagina can fertilize the egg in the fallopian tube. The fertilized egg begins its journey to the uterus.
17 18 19 20 21 22 23
Day 17 If pregnancy has occurred, the embryo passes into the uterus. By this time the hormones have prepared the lining to provide nourishment for the embryo.
24 25 26 27 28
Day 29 (or first day of next cycle) If pregnancy did not occur, the decrease in the hormone levels causes the uterus lining to break up and bleeding begins (period starts).

The Follicular Phase

This phase begins immediately following the menstrual period. It is that golden time of the month when you probably feel great. It is that 10-to-14-day period following menstruation when any PMS symptoms are completely gone. During this phase, your body's goal is to develop one mature follicle containing one egg, which will then be released from the follicle at the proper time.

Each ovary contains thousands of eggs, and almost all of these eggs are contained in tiny individual cystic areas called *primordial follicles*. At the onset of puberty there are approximately 300,000 eggs in a girl's ovaries, each in its own primordial follicle. During a woman's reproductive years, for every egg she releases (usually one monthly), there will be a thousand eggs that will not grow to maturity and will die that month. Except in the case of fraternal twins (or triplets, and so on), only one follicle grows to maturity for the day of ovulation. This one follicle is called the *dominant follicle*.

During the two weeks of its development, the dominant follicle produces increasing amounts of estrogen and releases it into the woman's body. This estrogen circulates in her bloodstream, flowing back around into the uterus, stimulating the uterine lining to develop in anticipation of a pregnancy. At the same time that the dominant follicle is producing estrogen, it is also filling with increasing

Presence of PMS Symptoms During Menstrual Cycle

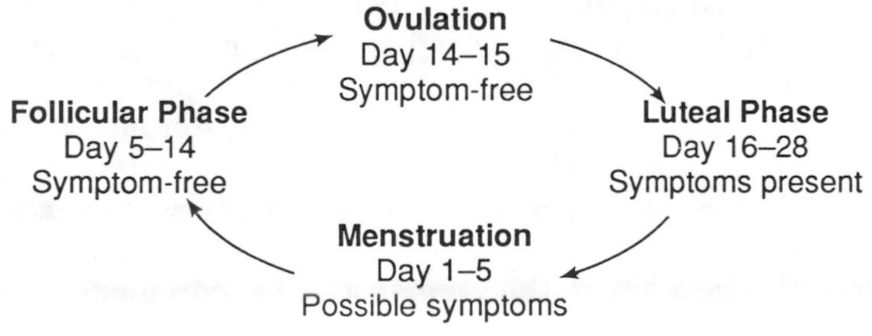

amounts of fluid. The egg is now maturing and being prepared for release from the ovary at ovulation.

The Ovulatory Phase

The purpose of ovulation is the release of the mature egg out of the ovary so that it can be picked up by the *fallopian tube* and eventually conveyed to the uterus. The actual process of ovulation begins as the outer wall of the follicle becomes thin and stretched and the amount of fluid in the follicle increases. Hormones called *prostaglandins* increase in quantity in the follicular fluid and in some way cause the follicle to rupture. Additionally, contractions of muscle cells in the ovary apparently cause both the fluid in the follicle and the egg to be squeezed out of the ovary. The rupture of the follicle and release of the egg from the ovary take only a few minutes. When follicle rupture occurs, the cystic fluid and the mature egg pass out of the ovary and are picked up by the fallopian tube.

Although the above process doesn't seem too terribly complicated, there are many hormonal processes going on simultaneously. At the end of the follicular phase, just before ovulation, there is a great deal of estrogen being secreted by the follicle which stimulates the pituitary gland to release a large amount of *luteinizing hormone* (LH) over a period of a few hours. Ovulation (release of the egg) occurs thirty-eight hours after this surge of LH reaches its peak. The empty follicle that once nurtured the mature egg now becomes the corpus luteum, which plays a vital role in both the reproductive process and in PMS. The corpus luteum begins producing progesterone, the hormone that completes the process of preparing the lining of the uterus for pregnancy. Progesterone will be released into the body's circulatory system and returned by the blood to the uterus to do its preparatory work. Even though progesterone is vital to a healthy pregnancy, it may also be a key to the premenstrual syndrome. As previously noted, many researchers feel that the changes that occur after ovulation, when progesterone levels are on the rise, are the true cause of PMS symptoms.

Luteal Phase

During the luteal phase, the lining of the uterus is prepared for an impending pregnancy. To accomplish this, the ovary secretes large amounts of progesterone and estrogen. Not only does progesterone participate in preparing the uterine lining for implantation of the embryo, but it also does other things, such as suppressing the ovaries to prevent other follicles from developing until the next menstruation. That too is vital to the maintenance of a healthy pregnancy. As the luteal phase begins, the cells lining the inside of the follicle remain after the egg passes out of the follicle. These cells are called *granulosa cells.* Other cells, called *theca-lutein cells,* may participate in the formation of the corpus luteum, which is responsible for production of both progesterone and estrogen. After ovulation, the granulosa cells change their appearance, developing a yellowish color. The theca-lutein cells become part of the corpus luteum and begin production of estrogen and progesterone. This hormone production peaks eight days after ovulation and begins declining during the next two or three days.

If pregnancy does not occur, the corpus luteum begins to degenerate, with a subsequent marked decrease in the production of progesterone and estrogen. When the degeneration is complete, a menstrual period will start. The luteal phase normally lasts fourteen days after the day of ovulation.

Menstruation

The major reason for menstruation is to rid the uterus of the lining it has built up during the previous fourteen days. This allows the development of a new lining, which will be receptive to an egg fertilized the following month.

As previously noted, a menstrual period usually occurs from every twenty-seven to thirty days during a woman's reproductive life.

As the corpus luteum dies, it no longer produces estrogen and progesterone, and this is what initiates menstruation. When the serum levels of these hormones drop below certain levels, the vessels of the inner lining of the uterus go into spasm, stopping the flow of blood to the lining, which then dies and begins sloughing off. This is characterized as menstrual "bleeding." Menstrual flow is made up of both dead tissue (formerly the lining of the uterus) and blood from blood vessels that have relaxed. Some of the menstrual flow is also fluid that has oozed through the raw surface of the uterine wall when its overlying surface disintegrated. Menstruation usually lasts for three to six days, but it is also considered normal for a woman's flow to last only one day or as long as eight days.

PMS is usually not a problem during menstruation. As the hormone levels gradually decrease during the luteal phase, symptoms usually decline. Some women will continue to have a few symptoms through their period, but all symptoms should stop when the period is over.

When the menstrual flow ends, the lining of the uterus grows once more, in response to the increasing levels of estrogen that are the result of the next follicular phase of the cycle.

6

Talking with Your Doctor About PMS

You may already be established with a physician who can help you with your PMS. If you are confident that your current doctor accepts the reality of PMS and is knowledgeable about its treatment, he or she would be the best consultant. Your existing patient/physician rapport will be valuable as you discuss your PMS and establish a plan of treatment.

Choosing a Physician

If you decide to choose a new physician, the following guidelines may help:

1. *Choose your physician wisely.* Take time and care in selecting a physician for PMS treatment. If you avoid seeing a physician who does not "believe in" PMS, you will save yourself frustration and disappointment. Dr. Joseph F. Mortola recently said at the Gynecologic Update presented by the University of California's San Diego School of Medicine, La Jolla, "With premenstrual syndrome we are going to have to take a look at the whole person again" (quoted in *OB/GYN News,* April 1–14, 1987). You should

expect this type of approach from your physician during consultations about PMS.

2. *Consider an obstetrician/gynecologist or a board-certified family practitioner.* These doctors may be more receptive to the idea that PMS is a reality and possibly more knowledgeable in this area. In particular, ob-gyns have had specialized training in women's health. A board-certified physician is one who has passed a rigorous examination in his or her specialty of medicine. This is important, as it may indicate a generally higher level of skill, training, and continuing education. Other physicians, such as internal-medicine specialists and surgeons, may be very capable in their fields but are often uninformed about PMS.

3. *Ask for referrals.* Sources of information you might consider before setting up an initial appointment include your current family physician, friends, the local medical society, or PMS clinics in the area. You may want to call more than one doctor's office for background information, unless all of your sources point to one physician.

4. *Talk with the office staff.* You can usually get a lot of valuable information from the receptionist and, better yet, the nurse in any medical office. If they have been with the physician for any length of time, they will know if that physician is interested in treating PMS. They will also be able to tell you about his or her approach to PMS.

5. *Ask specific questions.* When talking to the physician or nurse, ask about the specifics of the treatment program. Do they know local professionals to whom they can refer you for counseling about diet, exercise, and emotional problems if necessary? What kind of drugs do they recommend as part of the treatment program? Does the doctor use natural progesterone therapy? You may want to add your own questions to this list as you read further.

6. *Don't be afraid to make a change.* If your present physician seems disinterested or uninformed about PMS diagnosis or treatment, don't be afraid to make a change.

It is much better to try for a second opinion in the early stages of your treatment than to continue to see a physician who doesn't seem to accept or understand your problem.

7. *Don't set your first appointment at the time of your PMS symptoms.* You may be very anxious and tense at this time. If you see the doctor when you are not having PMS symptoms, you will be able to more rationally discuss both your symptoms and the proposed treatment.

What to Expect While Visiting Your Doctor

1. *Expect the physician to give you time to discuss your symptoms.* Your doctor will want a complete medical history. It is not important that you recount every single symptom you are currently having (there may be many). The most important information is found on your three-month PMS calendar, so bring it with you. This calendar documents the time in which your symptoms are occurring as well as their severity. If you have not kept such a calendar, the doctor will probably ask you to keep one for three months, as we have suggested in chapter 4. Then you will return for evaluation after it is completed. Expect to be in your doctor's office for an extended period of time on your first visit. This will allow adequate time for a discussion of your PMS calendar and symptoms and also for a review of potential treatment options. If the doctor rushes you and does not allow time for a thorough discussion, you may wish to seek another physician after your first visit.

2. *Expect careful observation by your physician before he or she arrives at a diagnosis and treatment plan.* Remember, your physician has not been living with you and has not seen your cyclic changes over a period of time. Almost half the patients who come to physicians seeking help for PMS have other problems instead. Your doctor will be trying to separate your PMS symptoms from pos-

sibly overlapping health problems, including emotional disturbances, psychiatric illness, and certain organic conditions, any of which may not be PMS-related. Time to make a diagnosis is needed, so be a patient patient! Don't push the doctor for a diagnosis he or she is not yet able to make.

3. *Expect your physician to ask many questions.* Not only will a medical history be taken, but many other questions will also be asked. Be prepared with the answers wherever possible. Things your physician will be interested in might include:

How are you feeling in general?

Have you seen other physicians concerning PMS? If so, what did they say? What specific treatments were tried?

What are your exercise and eating habits?

What do your responsibilities at home and at work entail? How are your relationships with family, workmates, and friends? What are your major sources of stress? Do you have unresolved conflict in your life? (These are important things for your doctor to know, since PMS and stress are so closely tied. Don't hold back. Tell your physician the full story in all these areas).

What are your menstrual cycles like? How long are your periods; how much do you bleed; do you cramp or not; are your periods regular?

Have you taken birth-control pills? If so, for how long and what kind? Did you notice any change in your PMS symptoms when you started or stopped taking the pills?

How did you feel just before and after you started menstruating during adolescence? Have those feelings changed over the years? How did you feel shortly after delivering a child and after your periods resumed following the cessation of breastfeeding? Have you ever thought that you might have had "postpartum blues"? (These are all times of great change in female-hormone levels, and for women with PMS they can be times of increased irritability and ill feeling.)

Do you have any chronic illnesses (such as arthritis, diabetes, lupus erythematosis) or other medical problems?

4. *Expect a complete physical exam.* This exam should include your heart, lungs, abdomen, pelvis, and, of course, blood pressure and weight check.

5. *Expect lab tests.* Tests ordered will vary with different physicians. Many doctors would normally order the following:

Complete blood count (CBC)

Complete urinalysis

SMAC 21 (a battery of 21 tests, which indicate the blood-sugar level, liver and kidney function, and other factors)

T3, T4 tests (for determining thyroid function)

Prolactin (if indicated by nipple discharge or irregular periods)

PAP smear (if you have not had one in the last twelve months)

You will notice that none of these tests is specifically indicative of PMS. You may ask why the doctor will not simply order a blood test to show whether or not you have PMS. The answer to this question is that there is no blood test that can diagnose PMS. It was once thought that abnormal progesterone levels might indicate PMS, but further investigation has revealed that there is no difference in serum progesterone for PMS and non-PMS women. Checking progesterone levels has absolutely no value for making a PMS diagnosis.

6. *Expect a diagnosis after a complete work-up.* After the lab work, physical exam, and three-month PMS calendar has been evaluated, you can then expect your physician to sit down with you and discuss whether or not your problems are caused by premenstrual syndrome. If you do have PMS, you should also expect a discussion of your treatment program at this time.

7

Accepting Your PMS Diagnosis

Women who seek a physician's care, receive a diagnosis of PMS, and then accept the fact that they have PMS are better able to deal with their symptoms. Breaking that emotional barrier can be difficult, though. It is not easy to accept the reality of having a physical/emotional impairment every fourth week just because you happen to be a woman. The reality of a full-blown case of PMS can be a difficult pill to swallow, but genuine acceptance will be well worth the effort.

Some women are actually relieved to know that what they have is PMS. It can be good news to learn that one's problem is not a catastrophic or life-threatening illness. This is particularly true for a woman previously seen by a physician who does not "believe in" PMS and was told that there is nothing wrong (that her emotional and physical symptoms are "all in her head"). This points out how important it is to choose a physician who accepts the reality of PMS. Acceptance that you are one of many women with PMS and that you can deal with this problem are the cornerstones of your hope for feeling better.

Once you have accepted the fact that you have premenstrual syndrome, you must turn your attention toward treatment. You have been diagnosed and now must take responsibility for entering the treatment phase. You need this so that you can feel physically better and more confident about yourself. You need this to be a more effective person—whether as wife, mother, friend, or working companion.

To a large extent, the success of your treatment program lies in your own hands and not those of your family or physician. No one else can enforce your diet or exercise program. No one else can make you take your medication on schedule. No one else can make you curtail your appointments to relieve unneeded stress. Only you can do all of these things. But when you do them you will find that your improved health will have made all the self-discipline worthwhile.

It is not an easy task to make major lifestyle changes. We know how hard that initial month of exercise can be while your muscles and joints are protesting that unusual movement. We are aware that we are asking you to do some things that you may find unpleasant, at least at first. But we are absolutely positive that you will grow to love your new way of life. In your victory over PMS, you will function better, be kinder to your family, be more in control—and you will serve God more enthusiastically and effectively.

Two factors stand out as your key responsibilities:

1. **Take your treatment program seriously.** Be true to your diet plan and exercise routine. Freely consult your physician, nutritionist, and exercise specialist.

2. **Pray for healing and steadfastness during your treatment program.** Pray for God's wisdom to work through your physician. Pray for your family to gain understanding for you and PMS. Pray for increased control on what were once out-of-control days.

Part 3

Treating PMS

8
Treatment Options

You have now reached a very important part of this book—the treatment program. We believe that with the help of these suggestions and input from your own physician, you will effectively deal with PMS and be a happier and healthier person. Did you know that you have already completed the first part of any PMS treatment regimen? You have become informed, interested, and reassured that PMS is a real and common occurrence. That's number one on anyone's treatment list, but now that you more fully understand what you are dealing with, we will pursue some more active approaches for the treatment of PMS.

One further point needs mentioning before we move on to the treatment outline. Though we are confident that PMS is a physiological problem (which may cause psychological symptoms), we are unsure of its exact cause and therefore somewhat uncertain about how to best treat the symptoms. Many researchers and lay persons are in disagreement over which treatments really work, and a discussion of the controversies alone could fill another book. Please understand that we have reviewed volumes of the most current literature and have given our professional opinions of which treatment options have merit. Also, what works for one patient may not work for the next. There unfortunately seem to be no hard-and-fast rules for treatment at this time. In some cases, we advise you to pursue these treatment options on a trial basis in an attempt to distinguish which ones make a difference for you.

Ready for one more frustrating and confusing bit of information? Even though professional opinions about what works and what doesn't may vary, in reality the suggested programs for the treatment of PMS at specialized clinics and through private physicians are all very similar. In fact, if the physician you choose sets out a program that deviates very much from the ideas incorporated in this book, it might be wise to get a second opinion. Above all, beware of so-called health professionals who promise a miracle. The miracle may be how quickly your wallet gets empty and how little your health gets better.

To acquaint you with an overview of the treatment options we recommend, we have made the following list. These options will be discussed in detail in subsequent chapters. The topics are divided into (1) suggestions that you can work on yourself, and (2) suggestions that will require your physician's care and supervision, including the use of prescription medications. Concentrate on the self-help chapters. Give them an honest effort. Keep a positive attitude, remembering that this syndrome can be dealt with. But don't overlook the help a physician and medication can provide if exercise, diet, and so on, do not give relief.

Things You Can Do Yourself

Education and reassurance
Pursue a regular exercise program
Maintain correct body weight

- Choose a correct diet
  - PMS diet plan (for days when you have PMS symptoms)
  - Regular diet plan (for other days of the month)
- Educate family and friends about PMS
- Make lifestyle changes to accommodate PMS days
- Control your stress
- Take vitamin and mineral supplements that may help PMS

Treatment Requiring a Physician's Supervision

- Correct diagnosis
- Elimination of other medical problems
- Referral to other professionals
  - For psychological help
  - For nutritional help
- Prescription medications as needed
  - Non-hormonal medications, such as diuretics and anti-anxiety preparations
  - Hormonal therapy
- Over-the-counter medications (get medical advice before using these)

9

Exercise and PMS

Although exercise may not cure your PMS, clinical studies show that a consistent exercise program will improve your general health and sense of well-being and can help control PMS symptoms (Prior and Vigna 1987; Prior, Vigna, and Alojada 1986). Consequently, we recommend a lively aerobic exercise program for almost all our PMS patients. Patient response to a consistent exercise program range from almost no effect to complete control over most PMS symptoms through exercise alone. This mode of therapy seems particularly helpful for those patients with extreme premenstrual stress. Since stress makes PMS worse, and exercise helps relieve stress, there is immediate benefit to one who suffers from PMS if she exercises. If you are not willing to exercise, it may be necessary for you to take increased amounts of medications for control of PMS. Even then, you still may not achieve your full treatment potential if you do not exercise.

Physiologically speaking, the benefits of exercise can in part be attributed to the release of *endorphins,* your body's "natural morphine" (or endogenous opiates), which accompanies rigorous and consistent exercise. These naturally-occurring endorphins, which are secreted by one's body during exercise can provide a mood elevation to your emotions and thus can improve your symptoms of PMS.

Both of us feel quite strongly that exercise is a significant component in the solution to the PMS problem for many women. Unfortunately, in this modern world in which we live, it is possible to get by with far less physical activity than our bodies were created to require. Because of this, many people who are not regular exercisers, do not feel as well as they could.

How Exercise Can Reduce PMS Symptoms

Every major publication about PMS that we researched included exercise as an important part of the treatment program. To be even more specific, it was aerobic exercise that was recommended. Some of the physical improvements that have been noted to accompany a long-term aerobic exercise program include the following:

1. *More Energy*. Decreased energy levels are a common complaint of many PMS women.
2. *Greater Productivity*. The inability to make decisions and the presence of fatigue can dramatically lower productivity in school, the work place, or home. Exercise helps this.
3. *Decreased Appetite*. Increased appetite and various food cravings are very common symptoms of PMS. Exercise can help reverse this.
4. *Reduced Stress*. A moderate amount of stress in our lives is normal and healthy. However, if we are in poor physical condition, even a small amount of stress may feel excessive. Physical conditioning can make a big difference.
5. *A More Positive Attitude*. This may be attributed to endorphin secretion, which can accompany an aerobic exercise program. Some researchers feel that PMS may be caused by the endorphin deficiencies that may occur premenstrually.
6. *Improved Ability to Handle Sugars*. Exercise enables the body to handle sugar in a healthier way, with

fewer peaks and valleys in the blood-sugar level. This can decrease the hypoglycemic feelings that many women have premenstrually.

7. *Decreased Body Fat and Improved Weight Maintenance.* There are suggestions that normalization of body-fat levels will also normalize levels of certain hormones, which may improve PMS.

A recent study in the *European Journal of Applied Physiology* has shown very encouraging preliminary data to support the thesis that exercise specifically reduces many common symptoms of PMS (Prior, Vigna, and Alojada 1986, 349). To paraphrase the researchers' summary notes:

> Conditioning exercises decreased premenstrual symptoms during a three-month study. Eight women with normal menstrual cycles began a walking/running exercise program while completing questionnaires about their PMS symptoms. Six other women followed the same program for three months but did not exercise. The PMS symptoms did not change in intensity for the sedentary group, but substantially improved for the exercising group. Specifically, breast tenderness, fluid retention, and general PMS symptoms decreased in the group that exercised.

Your Personalized Exercise Program

One thing is absolutely essential in selecting an exercise program—choose only activities you enjoy doing. It can be as simple as going out your front door and walking/jogging in your neighborhood for thirty minutes per day. It might mean setting up a stationary bike in your house or purchasing an exercise cassette or videotape to keep your program going during bad weather. Or you might choose a combination of all of the above so you don't get bored with any one program. You don't necessarily have to join a health club or organized community program, though you might enjoy it as a way to get moral support.

The main thing *is* to enjoy it! Be positive and happy about this decision. Dread will kill the program. Above all, remember that because you have made this decision, you will probably have a longer life and healthier, happier, and more productive days, with fewer PMS symptoms.

Question 1: How Do I Begin?

The chart below takes you from a novice program (for those who haven't exercised in years) through an advanced program. Be patient with yourself. If you need to start with the Week #1 program, be impressed with yourself for doing something. If you are currently involved in an exercise program, jump in at the level that seems appropriate. The key is consistency. The natural human tendency is to start above your physical capabilities, absolutely punish yourself for two weeks, and then give it up. Don't follow this pattern. It's demoralizing and will make it more difficult to begin a program next time.

Question 2: How Long and How Often Should I Exercise Each Day?

By following the chart, you will start with a nominal ten minutes of walking per day and eventually progress to a forty-minute workout four times per week. The definition of aerobic exercise is an activity that increases your heart rate to training level (see next question) and keeps it there for at least twenty minutes. You are actually exercising the heart and lung muscles when you do aerobic exercise.

Observe the following important suggestions throughout your program:

1. This is a suggested progression only. You should adjust the rate of your progress according to your own physical capabilities. *If you have health problems, consult your doctor before beginning.*
2. Always warm up and cool down. Any exercise session, even the ten-minute walks of the beginning weeks,

Progressive Exercise Program

Week	Duration	Frequency	Suggested Exercise
1	10 min.	7 times a week	Walking
2–3	10 min.	6 times a week	Fast walking
4	15 min.	5 times a week	Fast walking
5–6	20 min.	5 times a week	Fast walking
7–8	25 min.	5 times a week	Fast walking: 20 min. Calisthenics: 5 min.
9–11	30 min.	4 times a week	Walking or jogging: 25 min. Calisthenics: 5 min.
12 and after	40 min.	4 times a week	Walking, jogging, or aerobic dancing: 30 to 40 min. Calisthenics: 10 min.

should begin and end with a simple stretching routine: one or two minutes of stepping in place and reaching high overhead in an attempt to loosen your major muscles, especially in the legs, buttocks, and back.

3. At week #7 and beyond, the calisthenics should be done as soon as you finish your aerobic workout (fast walking, jogging, biking, aerobic dancing). Simple calisthenics, such as sit-ups, push-ups, leg-lifts and the like, are hard to beat. Do them at your aerobic exercising pulse rate without stopping between exercises. This will prolong your aerobic workout, help you with general muscle tone and condition, and increase your strength.

4. The suggested frequency pertains to the number of days each week on which you perform the activity. In other words, don't try to cram several sessions into one day to fulfill your goal for the week!

Question 3: How Hard Should I Exercise?

Assuming you are a healthy woman, with no medical history of heart disease (in which case you should definitely consult your physician for an exercise program), you can gauge the intensity of your exercise by determining your *exercising pulse rate*. Since you will need to time your ten-second pulse rate, we suggest that you purchase one of those great little $15 plastic exercise watches that have a second hand. For at least your first three months of exercise, you will have to take your pulse two times during each workout to determine if you are exercising at the suggested intensity for your age level. Follow the instructions below to find your appropriate exercising pulse rate:

(a) Find your pulse by placing your second and third fingers of your watch hand (usually left hand) on the underside of your wrist on the opposite hand, just below the crease. You must be able to see your watch (or another clock) as you count your pulses.

(b) After finding your pulse, count the number of pulses that occur in a ten-second period of time. Look at your watch carefully as you count. Be exact.

My 10-second resting pulse is____________

My 10-second exercise pulse rate range is ____________

(c) On the chart below, find your appropriate exercising pulse rate range according to your age.

Exercising Pulse Rates

Age	Pulse rate range for Aerobic Exercising (per ten seconds)
15	24–31
20	23–30
25	23–29
30	22–28
35	21–28
40	21–26
45	20–26
50	19–25
55	19–24
60	18–23

This is the range to which your pulse should increase to qualify as an aerobic workout. Whether you are jogging, walking, working out with weights, or even mowing your grass, your pulse (heartbeat) must reach the exercise pulse rate range stated above and stay there for twenty minutes for it to be considered aerobic exercise. *It is generally unwise to exceed this rate.*

Question 4: What Kind of Exercise Should I Do?

That's an easy question. Do what you like to do. In fact, it is essential that you find an exercise that suits you. The only stipulation is that it must be rigorous and consistent enough that your pulse rate stays up to exercising level for a full twenty minutes without dropping sporadically throughout the session. The best examples of aerobic exercise include walking, jogging, swimming, aerobic dancing, biking. This is certainly not an exhaustive list of aerobic activities. Even mowing your grass could be aerobic if you went at a fast enough pace and with no stops to move the garden hose.

Keep in mind that activities that require spurts of energy, such as tennis, basketball, football, water- or snow-skiing must be considered recreational and therefore should be done in addition to the regular aerobic workout. If your pulse falls below your exercising pulse rate range during your workout, it was not the best aerobic exercise.

Question 5: When Do I Start?

Nothing to do now but try the whole process—starting as soon as possible. Go out for five minutes or just walk or jog in place for a few minutes. At the end of this brief trial run, take your pulse. Is it higher than your resting pulse? Is it within the appropriate exercising pulse rate range? If it is lower than the suggested range, you will have to walk a little faster or in some way work harder. On the other hand, if your pulse exceeded the suggested range, you should slow down the pace of your exercise.

You should not exceed the rate range for your age unless you are in top condition and are getting professional help from an exercise physiologist.

Use the chart below to record your progress. You'll be amazed at how quickly you improve your stamina and strength. Enjoy it. Don't push yourself too hard. Look for small, consistent improvements each week or even each month.

Personal Exercise Diary

My favorite ways to aerobically exercise include: ______________

____

My aerobic exercise pulse rate range is from __________ to __________ pulses per 10 seconds.

Minutes of Aerobic Exercise per Day

Week No.	M	T	W	Th	F	Sa	S	Weekly Total
1								
2								
3								
4								
5								
6								
7								
8								
9								
10								
11								
12								
13								
14								
15								
16								
17								
18								
19								
20								

10

Diet and PMS

The role of nutrition in managing premenstrual syndrome has become an exciting new area of study. In a recent paper, Abraham and Rumley (1987) evaluated the clinical, biochemical, and endocrine effects of a total dietary program in patients with PMS. It was found that after PMS patients had consumed an improved diet for three to six months, their symptoms noticeably improved.

Three to six months? Yes, that's the long-term commitment for which you must be prepared before seeing any benefits from dietary changes. But your rewards will be long-lasting. Stay with it! Find new recipe books that make good-for-you foods also taste great. Think of this as a new lifetime attitude toward food—not something you do temporarily to make yourself feel better.

Reports about which nutritional changes are beneficial in the control of PMS are controversial. (Did you really expect anything else?) After consulting several references, we have compiled our own list of dietary changes that might improve your PMS. Though you should practice good nutrition habits throughout the month, the following rules are *most important during the last seven to ten days before your menstrual period begins.*

General Dietary Guidelines

1. *Eat well all month long.* Studies show that it is important to take care of your nutritional needs continually, as opposed to observing good nutrition in spurts. Accept the fact that most Americans eat a diet too high in calories, fat, and perhaps protein, while being deficient in fiber and other nutrients. (Instructions for an overall improved diet are included in this chapter.)

2. *Adjust your bodyweight if necessary.* It is probable that you may need to lose weight. This subject will be discussed below in detail. Meanwhile, let us say that being at your correct bodyweight will not only help you control your PMS, but will also improve your general health.

Premenstrual Dietary Guidelines

1. *Avoid sugars.* This includes table sugar, brown sugar, honey, molasses, jams, jellies, sugary drinks, or any other products made with large amounts of sugar or corn syrup. Hidden sugars are present in catsup, sweet pickles and relish, many breakfast cereals, and sweet mustards. Make use of artificially sweetened products during this time to satisfy your sweet tooth. If sugars are eaten premenstrually, this should be done in small quantities at the end of a meal. Avoidance of sugar will help you control the hypoglycemic reactions that are common in some cases of PMS.

2. *Avoid caffeine*—which is found in tea, coffee, many sodas, chocolate, and some aspirin-type preparations. Most PMS specialists make this recommendation which seems to reduce such symptoms as tension, anxiety, and insomnia.

3. *Avoid salt excesses.* That means limiting salty snacks, salted spices, and salty prepared foods. Beware of such condiments as soy sauce and Worcestershire sauce. Be light-handed with the salt shaker. Controlling your salt

intake will help you control water retention and bloating during the premenstrual days.

4. *Do not eat less than 1200 calories per day.* Premenstrually, you should certainly not overeat, but by the same token you should not undereat. Hypoglycemic reactions (tiredness, fatigue, lack of energy) may be worse if you are severely restricting your calories.

5. *Do not overeat.* More specifically, do not consume too many high-fat, high-calorie foods during the premenstrual time. This can add to a general feeling of lethargy and bloatedness.

6. *Eat more frequently.* It is advisable to eat five or six small meals per day premenstrually rather than three traditional meals. This essentially amounts to saving something from each meal and eating it two hours later as a snack. The Daily Meal Planner provided later in this chapter allows spaces for these snacks.

7. *Avoid alcohol.* It is reported that women are more sensitive to the effects of alcohol during their premenstrual phase. Use caution. It is probably advisable to avoid alcohol completely when you are premenstrual.

Adjusting Your Bodyweight

Our bodies seem to function so much better when we are at our proper weight, are exercising regularly, and are trying to make wise food choices. Unfortunately, the American lifestyle during the last four decades has been one that promotes the exact opposite of these healthy goals. Our lives seem to overflow with sedentary activities and excess stress, time-saving machines, and hi-fat, obesity-promoting foods. Fortunately, this trend is changing. People from every walk of life are now becoming aware that they must take responsibility for their own health. Preventive medicine has come of age.

When we prescribe dietary changes for patients, the

first procedure is to assess that patient's needs. Does she need to gain weight, lose weight, or maintain her current weight? We recommend that you find your ideal bodyweight range and adjust your current weight accordingly, if necessary.

In this section, we are specifically talking to women who require weight loss—not those of you who need to gain weight. The following are ways in which your PMS symptoms might be alleviated when you attain your appropriate bodyweight.

Improvement of Your Overall Health Status. Feeling healthier, more energetic, and less affected by health problems such as high blood pressure, heart disease, and diabetes will have a positive impact on your life. The increased energy you will feel should be especially important premenstrually.

Increased Self-Esteem. Low self-esteem is a significant problem with premenstrual women. Normalization of bodyweight will help relieve some of the anxieties rooted in a poor self-image.

Improved Carbohydrate Metabolism. Your body will be able to deal with sugars and starches more efficiently at your ideal bodyweight. As you probably know, hypoglycemia or at least hypoglycemic feelings are a significant problem for PMS women.

More Enjoyable Exercising. Let's face it. Exercise can be really tough if you are dragging around some extra weight. Trade that body-fat for muscle and you won't believe how energetic you will feel because of your increased basal metabolic rate (BMR).

Possible Normalization of Blood Levels of Some Hormones. Many women do not realize that obesity can affect their hormones in dramatic ways. There are higher estrogen levels in obese women than in women of normal weight, for example. (This may be the reason that obese women have a greater incidence of uterine cancer than thinner women.) Obese women are also more likely to have irregular periods and subsequent infertility. The long and short of it is that if PMS is even remotely connected to hormonal imbalance, your chances of controlling this syndrome will increase as your bodyweight normalizes.

Determining Your Ideal Bodyweight

How many times have you asked a doctor what you should weigh and received a range of weights varying by as much as twenty pounds for an answer? We want to help you pinpoint your ideal weight by showing you how to determine your true frame size. Then you can refer to the height/weight table provided in this book to determine your best weight. *A word of caution—don't guess at your frame size.* In our practices, we too often see thin people who think they have a small frame, while many overweight persons believe they have a large frame. This assumption is simply not true. Use the following steps to determine your true frame size (small, medium, or large) before proceeding to the height/weight table.

Determining Frame Size

To help you determine your own frame size, use the following calculations:

Your height in inches ____________.

Your right-hand wrist measurement just beyond (toward fingers) the little bone on the outside of your wrist in inches __________.

Height ÷ Wrist circumference = X

Determine frame size as follows:

female	male	frame size
X > 11.0	X > 10.4	small
X = 10.1–11.0	X = 9.6–10.4	medium
X < 10.1	X < 9.6	large

Your X value is ___________. Your frame size is ___________.

(Grant 1980, 15)

You are now ready to determine your own ideal body-weight from the height/weight chart below. You know your height and have just determined your frame size. Now find your ideal weight range, based on these figures.

Desirable Weights for Women
Age 25 or Over

Height (with shoes)		Weight in Pounds		
Feet	*Inches*	*Small Frame*	*Medium Frame*	*Large Frame*
4	11	95–101	98–110	106–122
5	0	96–104	101–113	109–125
5	1	99–107	104–116	112–128
5	2	102–110	107–119	115–131
5	3	105–113	110–122	118–134
5	4	108–116	113–126	121–138
5	5	111–119	116–130	125–142
5	6	114–123	120–135	129–146
5	7	118–127	124–139	133–150
5	8	122–131	128–143	137–154
5	9	126–135	132–147	141–158
5	10	130–140	136–151	145–163
5	11	134–144	140–155	149–168

For girls between 18 and 25, subtract 1 pound for each year under 25.

My *ideal* weight range is ______________________ .

My *current* weight is ______________________ .

I need to lose (or gain) ______________________ pounds.

The "Ideal Weight" Obsession

Let us say something more about "ideal weight." Far too much emphasis is placed on this single issue, especially by females. Women and girls of all ages are feeling the constant burden of keeping their weight or percentage of body fat at a level that may actually be too low for them. There is an endless barrage of "what we should look like" at every magazine stand, based on fashion-model standards. The result is an epidemic of anorexic/bulimic women who are so obsessed with weight control that they are paranoid about every mouthful and are often endangering their health. One further point, check some old Marilyn Monroe, Betty Grable, or Rita Hayworth photos. You'll find that these glamorous women still had a few jiggles—or, more scientifically, had a higher percentage of body fat than the models of today. Yet they were considered the ideals of physical beauty in that era. Clearly, it is difficult to take the ideal of the decade and alter your own weight up or down ten or more pounds without considerable physical effort and mental anxiety. Try to stay in your ideal bodyweight range, with the emphasis on *range*. Avoid body-type fads. Opt for health and vigor instead. Be happy with the real "you." God is.

The Meal Plan

In the previous sections, you have discovered (1) the ways in which proper diet may help PMS symptoms; (2) your ideal weight (versus your actual weight); and (3) the reasons why you should be at your ideal weight. All this information will help you deal more effectively with your PMS symptoms.

Two diet plans are given here to help you achieve these goals. They are very flexible and apply to both the premenstrual and postmenstrual times of your monthly cycle. Both are based on an exchange-system diet, wherein you are allowed a certain number of daily exchanges (or, for the most part, a certain number of servings) from each food group. Additionally, different calorie levels of each diet are given to help you with either weight loss or weight maintenance.

The regular diet plan should be used during times when PMS symptoms are absent—usually the first two to three weeks after your period starts. This diet can be used for either weight loss (at 1000- or 1200-calorie levels) or weight maintenance (at higher calorie levels).

The PMS diet plan is used during PMS times, usually the seven to ten days before your period starts. This can also be used for either weight loss (1200 calories) or weight maintenance (higher calorie levels). The PMS diet is slightly higher in protein and lower in carbohydrate than the regular diet plan, since hypoglycemic reactions are a common PMS complaint.

By using the regular and PMS diet plans at the appropriate times of the month, you will never wonder what you should be eating. Either diet should cover your needs at each stage of your progress. Remember, "diet" doesn't just mean weight loss; it means a plan for eating.

The Exchange Diet

Basic Concepts. The exchange-diet program is used as the basis for both the regular and the PMS plans. This concept has existed for many years and has weathered a barrage of "overnight success" diet schemes. It is also well respected among medical professionals for its many healthful benefits, including simplifying the idea of a "balanced diet." In recent years, it has been updated to include limited amounts of many popular items (hamburgers, pizza, etc.) and gives you limitless meal-plan options.

We will be changing the traditional exchange food lists, however, by reducing or eliminating foods of high fat content and/or low nutritive value. Our reasons for this are to help you prevent heart disease, breast cancer, uterine cancer, and some other things you don't want—but that is another story. It is sufficient to say that the diet provided here is oriented toward preventive medicine. Don't worry about an occasional piece of cake unless you eat it premenstrually. It's not what you do twice a month that matters, but what goes on daily.

Instructions for the Exchange Diet. There are six exchange lists in this chapter (pages 100-106) that will help you plan your meals. They include:

1. Starch/breads
2. Meats (includes fish and eggs)
3. Milk and milk products
4. Fruits
5. Lo-cal vegetables/free foods
6. Fats

In addition, there are sections that discuss combination foods and vegetarian diet plans. Foods are grouped together on a list because they are nutritionally alike. Every food on a list has about the same amount of carbohydrate (or fat or protein) and calories *in the quantities specified.* Therefore, they can be "exchanged" for any other food on the same list. Using the exchange lists and following the prescribed meal plans (that is, how many items on each list you can have per day) will provide you with great flexibility in your meals and snacks, optimal nutrition to promote good health, and enhanced blood-glucose control before and during PMS.

The following is a step-by-step guide to setting up your own diet plan.

1. Look at the table of "Regular Diet Plans" on page 95. This table should be used for the first two to three weeks after your period starts. If you are trying to lose weight, select the 1000- or 1200-calorie plan. If you are trying to maintain or gain weight, select one of the higher-calorie plans that you think best fits your caloric needs. If you find that it is not the right calorie level after trying it, choose another level later on.

2. Listed under the calorie plan you selected are the number of exchanges (or choices) from each food list that you are allowed each day. For example, if you choose the 1200-calorie plan, you are allowed four selections per day

from the starch/bread list and three from the fruit list. If you choose the 1800-calorie level, you may have eight starch/bread exchanges and four from the fruit list daily. Record these values in your "Daily Meal Planner—Regular Days" on page 96.

3. Make selections from the provided food lists to compile several daily menus for yourself using the calorie plan you have selected. Enter the selected food items on the "Daily Meal Planner—Regular Days" for this task, following the instructions and using the "sample" for reference.

4. "Extras" in your diet, including desserts, alcohol, and high-fat snack items not listed on the exchange lists may be eaten occasionally during the postmenstrual phase of your cycle. *Avoid these items when you are premenstrual, as they may increase your symptoms.*

5. When you are premenstrual, you should follow the same steps outlined above, except that you will use the "PMS Diet Plans" exchange list (page 95) and the "Daily Meal Planner—PMS Days" chart (page 98). In addition, refer to the special rules for PMS days at the beginning of this chapter.

Regular Diet Plans

Food Groups	Calorie Level				
	1000	*1200*	*1500*	*1800*	*2000*
			(No. servings/day)		
starch/bread	3	4	6	8	10
meat	4	5	6	7	7
milk	2	2	2	3	3
fruit	3	3	3	4	5
vegetables	3	4	4	4+	5+
fat	2	3	4	5	6

PMS Diet Plans

Food Groups	Calorie Levels			
	1200	*1500*	*1800*	*2000*
		(No. servings/day)		
starch/bread	3	4	6	7
meat*	8	8	9	9
milk	2	2	3	3
fruit	2	3	4	4
vegetables**	4	4+	5+	5+
fat	2	3	4	5

*Since so much meat (protein) is recommended in the PMS Diet Plan, it is very important that you choose the leanest choices possible. Baked, broiled, or poached chicken (no skin) or fish is preferable to beef or pork at this time.

**The symbol + indicates that you may have greater quantities of vegetables than the actual number of exchanges listed if you desire.

Daily Meal Planner—Regular Days

Instructions:

1. Choose a calorie level (1000, 1200, 1500, 1800, 2000)
2. Check "Regular Diet Plans" for the correct number of exchanges at the chosen calorie level.
3. Distribute the exchanges from all food groups throughout the day.
4. Check your food exchange list for correct food choices and quantities.

Sample Day (ex. 1200 cals)

	Number of exchanges	MENU	Number of exchanges	MENU Day____	MENU Day____	MENU Day____
Breakfast	starch 1 meat ____ milk 1 fruit 1 veg ____ fat ____	1/2 cup Raisin Bran 8 oz 1/2% milk 1/2 fresh banana	starch ____ meat ____ milk ____ fruit ____ veg ____ fat ____			
Snack	____ ____	(none)	____ ____			
Lunch	starch 1 meat 2 milk ____ fruit ____ veg 2 fat 1	2 pc. Life bread 2 oz. sliced turky Lettuce, tomato sprouts 2 tsp. Lite mayo	starch ____ meat ____ milk ____ fruit ____ veg ____ fat ____			
Snack	1 starch 1/2 milk	3-2 1/2 sq. graham crackers 4 oz. 1/2% milk	____ ____			
Dinner	starch 1 meat 3 milk ____ fruit 1 veg 2 fat 2	sm. baked potato Baked chicken breast 1/2 cup fruit 1 cup steamed veg 1 tsp. marg. 2T. Sour Cream	starch ____ meat ____ milk ____ fruit ____ veg ____ fat ____			
Snack	1 fruit 1/2 milk	1 peach 1/4 cup. low fat cottage Ch	____ ____			

	Number of exchanges	MENU Day____	MENU Day____	MENU Day____	MENU Day____
Breakfast	starch____ meat____ milk____ fruit____ veg____ fat____				
Snack	________ ________				
Lunch	starch____ meat____ milk____ fruit____ veg____ fat____				
Snack	________ ________				
Dinner	starch____ meat____ milk____ fruit____ veg____ fat____				
Snack	________ ________				

Daily Meal Planner—PMS Days

Instructions:

1. Choose a calorie level (1000, 1200, 1500, 1800, 2000)
2. Check "PMS Diet Plans" for the correct number of exchanges at the chosen calorie level.
3. Distribute the exchanges from all food groups throughout the day.
4. Check your food exchange list for correct food choices and quantities.

Sample Day
(ex. 1200 cals)

	Number of exchanges	MENU	Number of exchanges	MENU Day____	MENU Day____	MENU Day____
Breakfast	starch 1 meat 1 milk____ fruit 1 veg____ fat____	2 pieces Lite bread toasted 1 egg 4 oz. orange jc.	starch____ meat____ milk____ fruit____ veg____ fat____			
Snack	½ starch ½ milk	3-4 crackers ½ oz. skimmilk cheese	________ ________			
Lunch	starch____ meat 3 milk 1 fruit____ veg 2 fat 1	Lg. Chef Salad with 3 oz Lean meat 1 oz. skim cheese Lowfat Salad Dressing	starch____ meat____ milk____ fruit____ veg____ fat____			
Snack	½ starch ½ milk	3-4 crackers ½ oz skim milk cheese	________ ________			
Dinner	starch 1 meat 4 milk____ fruit____ veg 2 fat 1	½ cup cooked rice 4 oz baked or broiled fish 1 cup steamed vegetables 2 tsp. Low fat marg.	starch____ meat____ milk____ fruit____ veg____ fat____			
Snack	1 Fruit 1 vegetable	small apple carrot sticks	________ ________			

	Number of exchanges	MENU Day____	MENU Day____	MENU Day____	MENU Day____
Breakfast	starch____ meat____ milk____ fruit____ veg____ fat____				
Snack	________ ________				
Lunch	starch____ meat____ milk____ fruit____ veg____ fat____				
Snack	________ ________				
Dinner	starch____ meat____ milk____ fruit____ veg____ fat____				
Snack	________ ________				

FOOD EXCHANGE LISTS

#1: Starch/Breads

Items on the Starch and Bread list are approximately 70 calories per serving. Your most nutritious choices are those that are whole-grain products or are high in fiber.

Cereals—Grains—Pastas

bran cereals, concentrated	⅓ – ½ cup
bran cereals, flaked	½ cup
cooked cereals	½ cup
Grapenuts	¼ cup
other ready-to-eat unsweetened cereals	¾ cup
puffed cereals, unsweetened	1½ cup
flour, cornmeal, etc.	2 T.
rice, cooked	½ cup
pasta	½ cup
wheat germ	3 T.
(whole-grain varieties of rice and pasta are best choice)	

Crackers—Snacks

animal crackers	8
graham crackers, 2½-in. sq.	3
matzoth	¾ oz.
melba toast	5 slices
oyster crackers	24
popcorn, no fat added (no oil or butter)	3 cups
pretzels	¾ oz.
saltine-type crackers	6
whole-wheat crackers, no fat added	¾ oz.

Vegetables—Beans

beans, peas (cooked), such as kidney, white, pinto	½ cup
lentils	½ cup
peas, green	½ cup
corn	½ cup
potato, mashed	½ cup
potato, baked or boiled	1 small
squash, winter (acorn, butternut)	¾ cup
yam, sweet potato, plain	⅓ cup

Bread

bagel	½
bread sticks, crisp	2 (⅔)
bread, white or whole-grain	1 slice
lite bread, all varieties	2 slices
English muffin	½
frankfurter or hamburger bun	½
pita, 6-in. diameter	½
roll, small and plain	1
tortilla, 6-in. diameter	1
(whole-grain varieties are best choice)	

Breads Prepared with Fats

Note: Count these as one bread and 1 fat

biscuit, 2½-in. diameter	1
chow mein noodles	½ cup
cornbread, 2-in. cube	1
french fried potatoes, 2–3 in. long	10
muffin, very small, plain	1
pancake or waffle, 4-in. diameter	1
stuffing	¼ cup +
taco shell, 6 inch	1

#2: *Meats*

Each ounce of meat or meat alternative on this list contains approximately 7 grams of protein and from 55 to 80 calories, depending on the fat content. I have included the lean and medium-fat choices. Foods containing a very high fat content were excluded from the list, as they are not in keeping with a healthful diet.

Meat exchanges can be confusing. Remember, one exchange is not necessarily a normal serving size. In general, one exchange is one ounce of meat or the appropriate amount of a meat alternative, such as poultry, fish, eggs, and so on. Certain cheeses are included both here and on the milk and milk products list. If you count the cheese as a "meat" exchange, do not also count it as "milk."

Lo-Fat Meat Exchanges

MEAT	
lean beef (esp. round, sirloin, tenderloin) with no visible fat; lean pork or ham; lean veal; venison	1 oz.
POULTRY	
chicken, turkey, cornish hen (no skin or fat)	1 oz.
FISH	
any fresh or frozen (not fried)	1 oz.
crab, lobster, scallops, shrimp	2 oz.
tuna (canned in water only)	¼ cup
oysters	6
CHEESE	
any cottage cheese	¼ cup
Parmesan Cheese, grated	2 T.
special lo-fat cheeses (less than 55 cal/oz.)	1 oz.
MISC.	
egg whites	4 whites
Egg Beaters	¼ cup
95% fat-free lunch meats	1 oz.

Medium-Fat Meat Exchanges

MEAT	
ground beef, roast, porterhouse and T-bone steak, meatloaf; pork chops, pork loin, and pork roast; lamb	1 oz.
PORK	
most pork products, except sausage and bacon	1 oz.
POULTRY	
chicken *with skin*, duck, goose, ground turkey	1 oz.
FISH	
tuna (canned in oil, drained)	¼ cup
salmon (canned)	¼ cup
CHEESE	
Skim or part-skim-milk cheese, such as ricotta, mozzarella, and "diet" cheeses	1 oz.
MISC.	
Whole eggs (no more than 3 per wk.)	1
Tofu	4 oz.
Organ meats (high cholesterol!)	1 oz.
Peanut butter (high fat!)	1 T.

#3: Milk and Milk Products

If you haven't already made that switch to skim or lo-fat milk, resolve to do so now. Adults don't need milk fat. In this diet plan, we are counting on you having no higher than 1% lo-fat milk. There are just a few foods on this list. Dairy products high in fat are included in List #6.

We include cheese on this list for those women who cannot tolerate liquid milk for one reason or another. If you count cheese as one of your milk exchanges, do not count the same piece of cheese as meat in your menu planning.

MILK	
skim, ½% or 1%	1 cup
lo-fat buttermilk	1 cup
evaporated skim milk	½ cup
dry nonfat milk	⅓ cup
YOGURT	
plain, nonfat	1 cup
CHEESE	
lo-fat cottage cheese	½ cup
part skim cheeses	1 oz.

#4: Fruits

Each item on this list contains about 60 calories in the quantity specified. Be extra careful about the quantities, because they do differ. However, if something is not on the list, you may consider one fruit serving to be: ½ cup fresh fruit or juice, or ¼ cup of dried fruit. (When using canned fruit, choose "lite" or no-added-sugar varieties.)

FRESH (OR CANNED)	
apple, medium	½ apple
applesauce, unsweetened	½ cup
apricots, raw, medium	4 apricots
canned	½ cup
banana, 9 inch	½ banana
berries	¾ cup
cantaloupe, 5 in. across	⅓ melon
cherries, raw, large	12 cherries

fruit cocktail	½ cup
grapefruit, medium	½ fruit
grapes	15 grapes
kiwi	1 kiwi
orange, 2½ in.	1 orange
peach, 3 in.	1 peach
pear, large, raw	½ pear
pineapple, raw	¾ cup
canned	⅓ cup
plum, raw, 2 in.	2 plums
strawberries, fresh	1¼ cups
tangerines, 2 in.	2 tangerines
watermelon, cubed	1¼ cup
DRIED FRUITS	
apples	4 rings
dates	2½
prunes	3 medium
raisins	2 T.
FRUIT JUICES	
apple, grapefruit, orange, pineapple	½ cup
cranberry, grape, prune (higher in sugar)	⅓ cup

#5: Lo-cal Vegetables and Free Foods

This includes all non-starchy vegetables, such as asparagus, bean sprouts, greens, broccoli, brussels sprouts, cabbages, cauliflower, celery, cucumbers, carrots, eggplant, green beans, lettuces, mushrooms, okra, peppers, radishes, sauerkraut, spinach, summer squashes, tomatoes, zucchini, and onions. Sauces, butter, or dressings which might come with these foods should be a part of your alloted fat exchanges.

Seasonings that do not include sugars or large amounts of salt may be used as you wish, as may tea, coffee, sugar-free sodas. However, caffeinated products should not be used premenstrually except in very limited quantities.

#6: Fats

Items on this list include foods that are entirely composed of fat (i.e., butter) and items with such a high fat content that they are almost all fat (i.e., bacon, avocado, cream cheese). Each serving contains approximately 5 grams of fat and 35 to 45 calories.

If you want to avoid the trouble of counting fat exchanges, just use as little of these items as possible and use reduced-calorie or reduced-fat products, including diet margarine, lo-fat mayonnaise, and salad dressings with little or no oil.

CONCENTRATED FATS	1 tsp.
oil, butter, margarine, mayonnaise, salad dressings	
LO-FAT ALTERNATIVES	
reduced-calorie margarine	2 tsp.
reduced-caloric mayonnaise	2 tsp.
reduced calorie salad dressings	1–2 T.
NUTS	1 T.
OTHERS	
avocado	⅛ medium
olives	10 small
bacon	1 strip
coconut, shredded	2 T.
non-dairy creamer	1 T.
cream, light	2 T.
cream, sour	2 T.
cream, heavy	1 T.
cream cheese	1 T.
cream cheese, light	2 T.

A Note on Combination Foods

In general, you must learn to use your own judgment about combination foods such as casseroles, pizza, soups and stews, and the like. The best rule of thumb if you are cooking at home is to use only nutritious, non-processed ingredients. Examples are listed below:

Food	*Amount*	*Exchanges*
Pizza	1 slice (12″ pizza)	1 starch, 2 meat, 1 fat
Casserole	1 cup	2 starch, 2 meat, 1 fat
Chicken/vegetable soup	1 cup	1 vegetable, 1 meat
Cheeseburger	aver. size	2 bread, 3 meat, 1 milk
Chicken-vegetable stir fry	1½ cup	2 vegetables, 3 meat

A Note on Vegetarian Diets

Vegetarian diets work well in any balanced dietary program. The PMS diet program is certainly no exception. If you are a serious vegetarian, you should consult at least two good references on the subject to plan a nutritionally sound diet for yourself and your family. In general, make vegetarian substitutions (meat alternatives) for all the meat exchanges and keep everything else the same. Meat alternatives include cheese, eggs, tofu, soy protein products, beans and certain other vegetable combinations.

11

Drugs and PMS

Education, an active exercise program, and good dietary habits may be the only treatment program you need to control your PMS symptoms. You may, however, require more help to feel fully functional and happy during those difficult premenstrual days. Don't be ashamed of this need. Above all, don't focus on it as being an inherent weakness. Instead, be glad that there is something available that can help you control your premenstrual problems. The result can be a more productive, patient, and loving "you" all month long.

It is very important for you to be personally aware of the beneficial and detrimental effects of specific medications. As you read through this discussion of vitamins, minerals, and various drugs and their relation to premenstrual symptoms, you will understand why and how they are sometimes recommended. This will help you and your physician make wise choices for your own treatment program.

We do not recommend that you start by taking several medications at once. In general, it is preferable to start with at most one or perhaps two medications and see what they do for you. Otherwise, how could you possibly determine which of the new drugs helped you out? Try one at a time to get the best results.

The goal in this phase of the treatment program is to decrease PMS symptoms to a comfortable level. Few women are able to totally eliminate premenstrual symptoms. Through the combined effects of your total program though, you can be almost as comfortable premenstrually as you are postmenstrually.

Non-Hormonal Medications

Antiprostaglandins (nonsteroidal [not cortisone containing] anti-inflammatory drugs)

This seems like an intimidating name for such familiar products as Advil, Motrin, Anaprox and Ponstel. Recent studies have shown that these can be very helpful to women with premenstrual syndrome. They have widespread practical use, and we now use them as the first drug of choice for women with PMS. Two additional benefits include the fact that they are inexpensive and can be started just prior to the onset of PMS symptoms rather than be taken all month.

Some of the drugs in this group are over-the-counter preparations, such as Advil (ibuprofen) or even plain aspirin, while most of the others are by prescription only. In the past, this group of drugs has been used primarily to treat arthritis, but within the last decade has been used for treatment of dysmenorrhea (painful menstruation) and many other problems. In relation to PMS, it is hypothesized that antiprostaglandins, in addition to other functions, actually decrease the body's production of prostaglandins, thereby decreasing contractions of the uterus, gastrointestinal tract, and blood vessels.

Drugs in this category should be taken according to recommended dosages and/or in accordance with your physician's instructions. Ponstel, for example, can be taken as a 500 mg first-dose and then 250 mg every six hours thereafter. It should not be used for more than ten days of the menstrual cycle and seems most effective if begun a day before the expected time of the PMS symptoms. It should be continued until menstruation begins. Additionally, if you have cramping with your period, you should continue it for a few days after your period starts to help with the cramps.

If one of these drugs does not help, you may want your physician to try you on another. If two or three of them do not work, this is obviously not the solution for you and your own PMS.

There can be side effects from this group of drugs. For example, if you develop diarrhea while taking these medications, you should decrease the dosage or temporarily stop taking them. You should not use these drugs if you think you are pregnant or if you have kidney disease, intestinal ulcers, or inflammation of the intestinal tract. It is also important for you to know that if you take these drugs consistently for months on end, there can sometimes be detrimental effects on your liver. Remind your doctor that you are still taking them each time you return for your annual exam. He or she may want to run blood tests to assess your liver function.

Parlodel (bromocriptine)

This drug is frequently used for patients who have certain problems with their pituitary gland. This drug, however, is also very effective with patients whose major complaint with PMS is breast pain. Since most patients do not have breast pain of serious magnitude, we use this medication somewhat infrequently.

The drug is simple to use and is without any significant danger. The major side effect is that it can cause nausea to such an extent that patients cannot take a full dose or must discontinue use completely due to the gastric upset.

If breast pain is one of your major PMS complaints, ask your doctor about this drug. He will probably be comfortable in giving you a prescription. Dosages are usually

2.5 mg twice daily, one tablet in the morning and one in the evening.

Anti-anxiety Medications

Anti-anxiety medications (tranquilizers) are somewhat frowned upon in our society because of their overuse and misuse. That is unfortunate, because a judicious utilization of this group of medications can be very helpful. Our feeling is that if you have a medical problem that can be successfully treated by the moderate use of these drugs, you should try them under medical supervision. Only occasionally do we advise this as the first course of treatment. We usually recommend that you try dietary and exercise changes initially, and perhaps some of the other medications already mentioned. If all this fails or doesn't relieve your PMS enough for you to live a normal, happy life, this type of drug could be a partial answer for you. There should be no shame, embarrassment, or guilt associated with the appropriate intake of anti-anxiety medication. (We stress this point because Christian women often seem reluctant to try this mode of treatment, even if advised by their physician that it could mean relief from PMS symptoms.)

If some of your major complaints include insomnia, irritability, and tension, medications such as Tranxene, Xanex, Valium, or Librium can be of great help. The usual recommendation is a very small dosage used the day your PMS starts and stopped when your period begins. The use of anti-anxiety medication *in appropriate quantities* up to ten days out of the month will not usually promote addiction. If your doctor gives you this type of medication for PMS symptoms, we advise you never to use them at other times of the month—not for tension, nervousness, insomnia, or anything else. Such use might lead to drug misuse. Many women find that in combination with improved health habits, a mild anti-anxiety agent is all the PMS treatment they need.

As already mentioned, dosages of these drugs for PMS

treatment are small. In using Xanex, for example, the usual dosage is 0.25 mg three times per day. Very few women ever need more than this amount, even though this is not a large dose of medication. If Valium is your doctor's preference, you will probably use 2.5 mg three or four times per day.

Interestingly enough, it has recently been found that these drugs may also help the depression and the physical aching and discomfort sometimes associated with menstrual periods. This, an unexpected result, is a welcome discovery.

Diuretics

If bloating is a specific part of your problem, diuretics will probably be useful in your treatment program. The diuretic most frequently used with PMS patients is Aldactone (spironolactone). The use of this diuretic decreases swelling and water retention and has been shown to relieve other PMS symptoms such as depression and anxiety to a certain extent (Vellacott and O'Brien 1987).

Since this drug should not be given to patients who have kidney disease, your doctor may order a blood test to determine both your blood urea nitrogen (BUN) and potassium (K) blood level. If you are healthy and have never had kidney disease, your doctor may feel this test is unnecessary. Your doctor will probably begin you on 25 mg of Aldactone three times a day, starting three days prior to the time you expect your PMS to start. Continue to use this drug until the start of your period, or, if your PMS symptoms persist, continue taking it during the first few days of your period.

Aldactone has not been approved by the FDA for the treatment of PMS, but it does seem to be a safe and effective drug to use for this purpose.

Vitamins and Minerals

You probably don't think of vitamins and minerals as "drugs." In fact, you may be wondering why this discussion of vitamin/mineral supplementation and PMS was not included in the previous chapter, where an improved PMS diet program is outlined. The reason is that in large quantities, such as those found in some supplement preparations, vitamins and minerals are no longer nutritional compounds but drugs. If a person takes large amounts of vitamins and minerals, the body must deal with these substances as a medication, not as a nutritional substance. It does this by excreting, storing, or metabolizing (breaking down) these extra quantities to avoid levels that might be toxic to the human body. Yes, we did say "toxic," because large amounts of vitamins and minerals can be unhealthy. Therefore, *more is not necessarily better* when it comes to vitamins and minerals. The few supplements that do seem to have some credibility for reducing PMS are listed below.

***Vitamin B_6* (pyridoxine)**

Some of our patients feel that vitamin B_6 helps to reduce their symptoms. In the scientific literature, only about half of the studies about vitamin B_6 indicate that there is any relief of symptoms with supplementation of this vitamin. (Norris 1984). Based on this conflicting data, we usually recommend that a patient try this for a few months at a reasonable dosage to see if it helps. Dosages above 150 to 250 mg per day have been shown to produce neurologic damage, such as numbness in the feet, hips, hands, and face. Though these symptoms are usually reversible, we now recommend a lower dose of pyridoxine such as starting with 50 mg a day for the first week and then increasing to 100 mg a day thereafter. Pyridoxine should be taken all month long, not exclusively on premenstrual days. If after three months you cannot detect any difference in your PMS symptoms, you should discontinue vitamin B_6 supplementation. More importantly, if you begin noticing some numbness of your feet, face, or other parts of your body, stop B_6 supplementation immediately and do not use it again.

A few other practical points concerning B_6 supplementation are appropriate here. This vitamin can be a gastric (stomach) irritant. If you develop nausea or abdominal pain from the B_6, even though you take it with a meal, you should discontinue its use. If you have been on birth-control pills for a long time, your body's stores of vitamin B_6 may be low. Thus, women who are currently on birth-control pills or have been on them in the past six months may benefit from taking vitamin B_6.

One final warning: The notion that massive doses of any water-soluble vitamin (of which vitamin B_6 is one) may be administered without bodily harm is absolutely false. Various scientific studies have clearly demonstrated the dangers of such massive dosage (van den Berg, et al. 1986). Be particularly careful of persons who are eager to sell you vitamin/mineral supplements but are not true health professionals. Although they have usually attended brief seminars given by the companies they represent, they usually do not understand the full picture.

Magnesium and Calcium

American women may have a deficiency of magnesium in their diets (Abraham 1983), and at least one recent study has recommended a magnesium supplement for women with PMS (Chihal 1985). Magnesium supplementation seems to decrease the chocolate craving experienced by some patients during PMS time. Chocolate contains a large amount of magnesium, and this may explain the craving.

It has also been recommended by some experts that women with PMS restrict their calcium intake because the presence of this mineral decreases magnesium absorption. We do not agree with this mode of therapy because osteoporosis (bone loss due to inadequate intake of calcium) is such a rampant problem for American women.

If you experience cravings for chocolate, magnesium supplementation might be helpful. The dosage we recommend is 250 mg a day, taken throughout the month. The best way to achieve a consistent dosage is to take a general vitamin/mineral supplement that also contains 250 mg of magnesium. The best food sources of magnesium include whole grains, green leafy vegetables, legumes, nuts, seeds, cereals, and shellfish. More importantly, some of the foods that contain the highest magnesium/calcium ratio include millet, corn, potatoes, wheat, and cashew nuts.

Evening Primrose Oil (Efamol)

Evening primrose oil (Efamol) has been advocated during the past few years for women with PMS. This drug seems to have no significant adverse side effects except that a few women have reported some skin blemishes while using it. A few studies have shown that women who have not responded to other methods of therapy will occasionally respond to the use of Efamol for PMS symptoms. This drug contains large concentrations of gamma-linolenic acid, a compound that is possibly used by a woman's body to make her less sensitive to a hormone called *prolactin.* Prolactin sensitivity may be one of the causes of PMS symptoms. Many women find that they must use evening primrose oil for two or three months before they feel relief from their PMS symptoms.

The usual beginning dosage schedule for the use of Efamol is two 0.5 mg capsules of Efamol twice a day (four capsules a day), starting as soon as ovulation occurs. If you are not helped by this dosage, gradually increase to four capsules twice daily, a total of eight capsules per day. Eventually you may be able to cut back this amount to four capsules per day, to be taken only on premenstrual days. Initially, however, to avoid an upset stomach this supplement should be taken daily with a meal for the first few months.

The evening primrose plant is a wildflower found in

North America, and the oil is found in the seed portion of the plant. The processed and bottled oil can be found in pharmacies and various health-food stores and is available without prescription. Be sure to read the label, since other so-called PMS oils may be next to it on the shelf. These other "PMS oils" may contain such foreign substances as dolomite (which contains lead) or may have unreliable levels of evening primrose oil in the capsules.

Progesterone—The Hormonal Treatment

The primary argument among physicians about the treatment of PMS with progesterone revolves around whether or not it really works. It is our feeling that *in certain cases* it does indeed work. Many, but not all, women have found that progesterone supplementation does help their PMS symptoms, and during the last few years some research studies have substantiated that finding.

One advantage of this drug is that it does not seem to have any severe side effects. Therefore, a woman can try it with negligible risk. Because natural, safe progesterones are used for PMS, we feel it is unlikely that the use of the drug presently will cause any future health problems.

One further point—*if progesterone does work for you, don't ignore other aspects of your personal program.* Dr. Katharina Dalton of Great Britain, one of the most ardent supporters of progesterone therapy for PMS over the last thirty years, advocates the use of progesterone, but states that the patient and physician must coordinate a total program—which includes diet, exercise, and many of the other things we have discussed in this book (Dalton 1984).

How Progesterone Is Used

If you were already aware that progesterone is sometimes used in the treatment of PMS, you may also have been aware that using natural progesterone is not as simple as popping a pill in your mouth. In fact, it is usually taken as a rectal or vaginal suppository or foam preparation to facilitate absorption of the drug. The form of progesterone recommended by physicians who treat PMS is natural crystalline progesterone, a very different product from the synthetic progestins. In the past, when the natural form was taken by mouth, it was broken down in the digestive tract before it had a chance of being absorbed. A new form of natural progesterone called *oral micronized progesterone* is now available for PMS treatment. Though it is used in the United States to a very limited extent, it has been found to be effective in relieving PMS symptoms. This form of progesterone may replace the vaginal and rectal progesterones (most women would say "gladly"). Your doctor can obtain this form of progesterone from:

Madison Pharmacy Associates
429 Sammon Pl.
Madison, WI 53719
1-800-558-7046

A practical note about progesterone suppositories is necessary. Unfortunately, these products are not made by any major drug company and must ordinarily be made locally by your pharmacist from a powder available from drug suppliers. This custom production does tend to make them expensive. A second disadvantage of the suppositories is that they can be messy. When inserted vaginally, they melt and then tend to run out of the vagina. If inserted rectally, they may intensify intestinal motility, which can result in increased gas and diarrhea. These side effects do not always occur, and you may have no side effects, so the main idea is to simply try them on your physician's recommendation. Give them a four-month chance to work. If they haven't helped by then, or the side effects outweigh the benefits, discontinue using them.

The usual dosage of progesterone suppositories ranges

from one to six 200 mg suppositories per day. About 10 percent of patients need to use only one suppository per day, but most patients will use two to four daily. Women should use the suppositories a day or two before their PMS symptoms are expected and continue use until the menstrual period begins. After having used the progesterone suppositories successfully for months, some women are able to discontinue this medication without the return of PMS symptoms. Other women, however, must remain on progesterone indefinitely to maintain PMS control.

If you want to try the oral micronized form, the dosage starts at 100 mg a day and increases to 300 mg a day. Medication should be taken on the same regime that is used for vaginal progesterone. This recommended dosage may change as more studies on its long-term use are conducted.

Another reminder: This form of progesterone will not work as a contraceptive. Remember, your PMS starts when one of your ovaries releases this month's egg. You could become pregnant the day your egg is released any month that you do not use contraceptives (or even occasionally if you do use contraceptives—no contraceptive is perfect). Since PMS starts after ovulation and medication is started after ovulation, pregnancy could occur any month. Also remember that if you did become pregnant, you would still have PMS during the two weeks before you missed your period. The hormones of pregnancy would not prevent PMS during those first two weeks. Therefore, you could be pregnant, have PMS, and be using medications for PMS all at the same time.

Natural progesterone would not harm your pregnancy—I use it in my infertile patients to help them maintain pregnancy. However, if you are taking other drugs for PMS, ask your doctor if they would endanger a pregnancy. If so, use careful contraceptives any month that you are taking those drugs.

Natural progesterone can be used rectally, and suppositories can be used vaginally. A more comfortable form, however, is liquid progesterone. The fluid is drawn into a syringe and inserted into the rectum. The fluid contains 200 mg of natural progesterone per cc and can be used according to the same schedule recommended for vaginal suppositories. An advantage to this treatment is that it eliminates irritation of the intestine, such as loose stools and increased gas, which may be a problem for you. The liquid form is also less expensive and not as messy as using the progesterone vaginally. This medication is available only by prescription.

There is one other potential side effect. For some women, the use of progesterone supplements can prevent their periods from starting. This is not dangerous but can be upsetting, especially if a woman is not sure whether or not she is pregnant. If your menstrual period is delayed, the progesterone can be stopped and a period would normally begin. If this side effect happens to you, discuss this matter with your physician.

Other Forms of Progesterone

There are synthetic progesterone formulations that can be used in conjunction with PMS. Though Katharina Dalton (1984) has stated that these synthetic forms do not help PMS patients, many individuals have found them to be helpful. These medications include Depo-Provera, a drug that can be given as an injection (150 to 200 mg) every three months. However, we do not recommend that a patient use this medication unless she does not want any more children. The drug can prevent a menstrual period for many months or can make a woman bleed every day for many months after she gets even one injection. It is nevertheless helpful to some women with PMS and is certainly less expensive than the natural progesterones. An additional benefit of Depo-Provera is that one shot provides contraception for three months.

Provera is an oral form of Depo-Provera, and many patients have found that taking Provera from two or three days after the time of ovulation until the time of the period—and then stopping it to allow the period to start—gives some relief from PMS symptoms. To know whether or not this drug would help you, you must simply try it (that is, if you fit the criteria already stated, and your doctor will prescribe it). Some physicians recommend using Provera in a dosage of 20 mg per day (by mouth) every day. This will eliminate ovulation as well as menstrual periods. Some patients do very well with this mode of therapy, while others may have breakthrough bleeding when they take Provera daily. On the other hand, some women will not have periods if they take Provera every day. If a woman doesn't mind the breakthrough bleeding or the lack of periods (whichever she has), it is fine for her to take Provera. Neither bleeding pattern is damaging. One important warning is that a woman cannot depend on Provera to provide contraception. If she becomes pregnant while using Provera, it can cause abnormalities in her child. Therefore, she must not get pregnant while she is using Provera.

Oral Contraceptives

Birth-control pills can help some women alleviate PMS symptoms. Again, the only way to know if they will help you is simply to try them. If you do not want to get pregnant at the present time, if you are below the age of forty, and if you have no other reason to avoid oral contraceptives, we recommend that you try them. Just remember that some people will become depressed and moody with these pills, but others have the opposite reaction. Also, if you are a smoker, you should not use birth-control pills over the age of thirty-five. Doctors have generally found that oral contraceptives will help about one-third of the women who use them to control PMS symptoms. One-third of the women reported no change in their symptoms, and one-third reported an increase in symptoms.

Other Medications

Danocrine (danazol)

This somewhat unfamiliar drug is used primarily for problems not related to PMS, such as endometriosis and breast pain and breast nodularity. The use of danazol in PMS is relatively new. The usual dosage for PMS treatment is 200 mg three times per day, beginning just before the start of symptoms and continuing until menstruation starts. If no other drug has been helpful for you, discuss this one with your doctor to determine if it might be a reasonable next step to try. *This drug is not a contraceptive, and it can cause abnormalities to your fetus if you use it while pregnant.*

Lithium

Lithium has been used with a few PMS patients, usually those who experience wide mood swings premenstrually. Remember that lithium is usually prescribed for patients with manic-depressive illnesses (psychological disturbances characterized by excessive mood swings). This drug would be recommended only if you fit this criterion and would probably be administered under the care of a psychiatrist. *You should not get pregnant while taking lithium.*

Gonadotropin-releasing Hormone Agonist (GnRH agonist)

This drug has been used for the treatment of PMS only in research studies. It may be used more widely in the future. It is generally used to stop ovarian hormone secretion and ovulation. In one recent study, it totally stopped PMS in a group of women (Muse 1984).

Since this drug actually puts the ovaries to sleep, keeping them not only from ovulating but also from producing estrogen and progesterone, this would not be a drug to use for a long period of time. When their ovaries are producing no estrogen, women are at risk of developing osteoporosis, dryness of the vagina, hot flashes, and other symptoms that mimic menopause.

Further studies are necessary to completely evaluate this mode of treatment and especially to evaluate long-term effects on women.

Synthyroid (synthetic T4)

Treatment with Synthyroid has proven useful in the treatment of some patients with PMS (Brayshaw 1987). The study that documented this was preliminary, however, and has not been validated by other researchers. It will be interesting to see if this drug will have an important place in PMS therapy.

Part 4

Living with PMS

12

Family, Friends, Lifestyle, and PMS

Educating Those Around You

Family and friends are often in the dark about a woman's trials with PMS. They often do not recognize the cyclic nature of family discord, marital stress, and workplace conflict. And, too often they will remember only the bad times and forget the good ones. If you have a diagnosed case of PMS, you owe it to yourself and your family to discuss it with them. They will almost immediately realize that there has been a cyclic pattern to your periods of irritability. They will also recognize that you do have good days—times when you are a different person than who you become on "those PMS days." This will enable them to accept the whole "you" and even encourage you as you start your new PMS treatment program.

Even though it may be difficult at first, be receptive to encouragement that can come from those you love, especially your family. In particular, your husband's encouragement might take the form of his being your exercise and/or diet partner, or he may help keep sweets and caffeine out of the house, at least when you are premenstrual. One last thing, keep a discreet PMS calendar in a convenient location, so that your husband can check the phase of your cycle without having to ask. Take heart—when you find the portions of the PMS treatment program that work for you, your body will feel so much better that there may be very little need for this calendar anymore.

The Right Time to Talk

There is a right time to talk about your PMS with family and friends. That time is during the week after your period is over, when you can see things most rationally and objectively. When you are already premenstrual, you may be reluctant to discuss it calmly with your family and will usually feel completely justified in your ill feelings toward them! It may seem as if the world is out to get you—especially the world in your own household. You may feel as if you are seeing things clearly for the first time in days—that this is the only time when you are really aware of your tough situation in life. Then, a week later, after your period is over, it will be almost like having amnesia. Are your children really that disobedient? Is your husband truly that bad a spouse? Is your job as lousy as you thought it was last week? Is your best friend really ignoring you? The answers to those questions are no, no, no, and no. There may be problems, yes, but they always seem blown out of proportion premenstrually. The lesson to be learned from this is to inform others about your PMS during the good days. You may be unwilling to do this while you have PMS and ineffective if you try.

A Special Note to Husbands

Give many hugs and kisses to your wife during her premenstrual days. It is very important that you realize that during her PMS time a woman may have a decreased sexual drive, coupled with lowered self-esteem. Therefore, husband, be generous with your tenderness and affection during the PMS time without expecting that your thoughtfulness will be rewarded (by sexual intimacy). This type of undemanding love will help your wife be less tense and will help improve her sense of self-esteem at this low point in her month. Many premenstrual wives refuse even simple gestures of affection from their husband because they know that he will expect to follow through to intercourse. And this they just do not feel like doing! The result is even lower self-esteem premenstrually fostered by a total absence of physical affection and a general feeling of estrangement from their husbands.

A Special Note to Wives

Since we gave a special note to husbands, we thought a special note to wives is in order. One of the potential traps you can fall into is using your PMS against your husband. It is all too easy to use it as an excuse for your anger and hostility toward him or as the reason for not getting your work done well or at all. You may misuse PMS as a measure of your husband's love and sensitivity—wielding it as a club if he is not understanding enough (by *your* standards) at your PMS time. You can so misuse your PMS that you cause your husband to leave you, emotionally if not physically, and drive your children away as well. Get help for your PMS. Treatment will make a difference. Don't hide behind your symptoms and thereby miss a lot of good living.

A Special Note for Mothers

Children are one of the greatest of God's blessings. But, let's face it, being a parent is not always easy. In families with more than one young child, your physical and emotional strength can literally be gone by noon. If you couple the normal physical drain of being a mother with untreated PMS, you may find effective and loving parenting to be an impossible hurdle on premenstrual days.

This became personally clear to Dr. Sneed one hot and

muggy summer afternoon in Texas before she began her own treatment program. This is how she remembers it:

> Those of you who are mothers can envision this scene, I'm sure—a hot car, a crying baby, an overly talkative six-year-old, a rambunctious three-year-old and a screaming, premenstrual mother. After the last excrutiatingly loud scream, it is suddenly quiet. Then the three-year-old says, "God doesn't like you to scream at us, Mommy," as big tears well up in her eyes. The child's best friend and greatest security had just betrayed her. Plus, she was right—God doesn't like all that screaming. The time for my own serious treatment had come. But how do you inform young children about PMS? The words I used were, "Mommy is sick today. I am very sorry for being unloving. I am going to try very hard to be nice even though I don't feel well. I love you very much."

Don't be afraid to apologize for poor PMS behavior. Just do your best to control things better next time around by being faithful to your treatment program and faithful to God in your prayer life.

A Special Note for Families

A household that has more than one menstruating woman may be in for a double or triple dose of PMS. When two or more women live together, they tend to start menstruating at the same time. No one knows what causes this to occur, but there is evidence that women who live together often experience their PMS at the same time. This same phenomenon can occur in a dormitory situation, in a house with several women rooming together, or perhaps even in an office.

There are two obvious results of this. First, the women with PMS must interact with each other when they are least able to be rational and objective. To put it more bluntly, they are dealing with each other when they are the most likely to be angry, quick-tempered, easily hurt, and withdrawn. Women in this situation should be open with each other concerning where they are in their cycles. If their cycles are coordinated, they should agree to avoid emotional interaction and controversy at PMS times.

The second obvious result of coordinated PMS cycles is that husbands, sons, fathers, and brothers can be caught in the crossfire. Just knowing what the problem is can help those who live in a household with "mass PMS." The considerate action for the women to take might be a gentle warning of things to come. Treatment of PMS should alleviate most of these problems, in any event. (Of course, it is rarely appropriate to discuss one's PMS symptoms with male co-workers, but some of the suggestions in the next section about "lifestyle" and in chapter 13 ["Stress and PMS"] might be applicable to your professional life.)

Adjusting Your Lifestyle and Schedule to Your Cycle

Live with your menstrual cycle. Don't fight it! In her book *The Joy of Being a Woman* (1975), Ingrid Trobisch suggests that women should be aware of the time they expect their premenstrual symptoms and reserve that time for the quiet activities of life, such as reading and doing things that do not require much interaction with other people. Obviously, you will have to adjust your schedule according to your responsibilities and the severity of your PMS symptoms. A few of you may have to call a brief halt to some activities, while others will benefit from only a slight curtailment of their schedule.

Why is this important? It is probable that PMS is aggravated by even minor outside factors that cause additional tension. That is, what normally might be a slight problem may become a huge, anxious dilemma during PMS time. Carefully schedule your activities as you work toward the control of your PMS. Once your PMS is under control, you can experiment with your schedule to see how much stress you can tolerate at that time. If your PMS does not seem aggravated by a month-long full schedule, you probably do not need that constraint any longer.

Here are some practical ideas that might be helpful while your PMS is being brought under control:

1. Avoid social commitments that are personally demanding, such as dinner parties or other gatherings that require you to be responsible for elaborate preparations.
2. Be more productive during other parts of your cycle so that you can take more time to relax when premenstrual.
3. Schedule vacations during the first two weeks after your period.
4. If possible, arrange car pools and other such commitments on a rotation that frees you from responsibility when you are premenstrual.
5. If you have young children at home, arrange for occasional baby-sitting during your premenstrual time. This is a tremendous aid to mothers, especially if they are dealing with PMS problems.

13

Stress and PMS

Stress. We all talk about it. We all think about it. We all seek ways to get rid of it. But how much do you personally know about what stress is and how it relates to premenstrual syndrome? Even though stress is an important part of our lives, we seem to know so little of its true nature. According to one dictionary, stress in humans is "a physical, chemical, or emotional factor that causes bodily or mental tension and may be a factor in disease causation; also, a state of bodily or mental tension resulting from factors that tend to alter an existent equilibrium."

In fact, PMS can be one of those "factors that tend to alter an existent equilibrium." Think of it this way—everyone has a few burdens that they must carry with them each day. Pretend that you can give them all a value in pounds and then put them in a pack that you carry on your back constantly. Let's say that though your level of stress, burdens, and cares certainly varies from day to day, the average value of your load is thirty pounds. That sounds like an amount that you can live with. Life might be easier without having to carry around thirty pounds of extra burden, but it is manageable. During the premenstrual time of the month, however, the added physical and emotional strains of PMS may double or triple the weight of that once-bearable load, creating a crushing albatross that could only be carried by Superman (or, in this case, Superwoman). A vicious cycle can develop, though stress does not cause PMS, it can increase premenstrual symptoms. Then, PMS can actually create new stress, and the increased stress can make PMS worse.

Some stress in life's happenings is absolutely necessary and productive. Since almost any responsibility involves some pressure, stress can actually help us complete our work on time. This book, for instance, would not have been written if we had not been willing to endure a certain amount of stress. If your stress level is excessive, however, it stops being beneficial and starts being detrimental and counterproductive. If you find that life's tensions and stresses are beyond your coping abilities, you may need to get some counseling to learn how to decrease your stress load and to help your PMS.

Recognizing Stress in Your Life

Stress may cause you to shake, to sweat, or to be unable to sleep. These and other physical signs of stress are a result of the excessive production of hormones from your adrenal glands. The overproduction of adrenal secretions can be caused by any event, positive or negative, that forces you to make changes in your life. We are aware that negative factors such as illness, poor interpersonal relationships, or difficult financial situations will cause stress. However, we rarely think of a job promotion, or the birth of a healthy child as being stressful—but, indeed they can be.

A classic stress-measurement test was developed in 1967 by Thomas Holmes and Richard Rahe, psychiatrists at the University of Washington School of Medicine. Their test, which is called the Social Readjustment Scale, rates the stressfulness of various life events from minimal stress (valued at 1) to maximal stress (valued at 100) (Holmes and Rahe 1967).

A copy of this stress test is below. Review the items and check off those that you have experienced within the previous twelve months. If your score reaches or exceeds 300, you are overstressed and have a 90 percent chance of becoming ill or having a major accident because of stress in your life. Keep in mind, using our backpack illustration above, that even a score of 100 to 200 may mean that you have enough stress during the premenstrual time of the month to make your PMS much worse. (*Note:* The dollar values have been changed to accommodate current inflation rates.)

Signs and Symptoms of Excessive Stress

Patients often inquire about the ways in which they can rate their ability to handle stress as normal or abnormal. Above all, if you are constantly feeling pressured or overburdened and becoming anxious or depressed for no significant reason, you may be handling stress poorly. This is particularly true if you are also dissatisfied with yourself or feel that you cannot cope with your present life.

There are many physical and mental problems thought to be associated with out-of-control stress. The following list is reprinted from *1250 Health-Care Questions Women Ask*. Look at this list honestly and determine whether (1) you suffer from these problems most of the time, or (2) whether they seem to occur more often or exclusively when you are premenstrual. (This list originally appeared in a 1984 article in *Philadelphia Magazine* [Los Angeles Times Syndicate]).

Motor tension. Shakiness, tension, aching muscles, inability to relax, jumpiness, or fatigue.

Uncontrollable body sensations. Sweating, pounding heart, clammy hands, dry mouth, dizziness, light headedness, hot or cold flashes, upset stomach, lump in the throat, diarrhea, pallor or flushed face.

Apprehensive expectation. Fear, worry, rumination, anticipation of misfortune to self or others.

Social Readjustment Scale

Life Event	Stress Value
Death of a spouse	100
Divorce	73
Marital separation	65
Jail term	63
Death of a close family member	63
Personal injury or illness	53
Marriage	50
Fired from job	47
Marital reconciliation	45
Retirement	45
Change in health of family member	44
Pregnancy	40
Sex difficulties	39
Gain of a new family member	39
Business readjustment	39
Change in financial state	38
Death of a close friend	37
Change to a different line of work	36
Change in number of arguments with spouse	35
Mortgage over $50,000	31
Foreclosure on mortgage or loan	30
Change in responsibilities at work	29
Son or daughter leaving home	29
Trouble with in-laws	29
Outstanding personal achievement	28
Wife begins or stops working	26
Beginning or end of school	26
Change in living conditions	25
Revision of personal habits	24
Trouble with boss	23
Change in work hours or conditions	20
Change in residence	20
Change in schools	20
Change in recreation	19
Change in church activities	19
Change in social activities	18
Mortgage or loan less than $50,000	17
Change in sleeping habits	16
Change in number of family get-togethers	15
Change in eating habits	15
Vacation	13
Christmas	12
Minor violations of the law	11

T. J. Holmes and R. H. Rahe, "The Social Readjustment Rating Scale," *Journal of Psychosomatic Research,* Vol. 11. Copyright 1967, Pergamon Press, Ltd.

Constant hyperattention. Difficulty with concentration that leads to irritability, impatience, insomnia, and the feeling of always being on the edge of panic.

The sudden onset of explosive, overwhelming feeling of terror. This is as if the body's alarm system were ringing for no apparent reason.

Unreasonable fear. Fear of flying, fear of closed spaces, fear of getting up in the morning.

Handling Stress

Dr. Holly Atkinson, former medical editor for "CBS Morning News" has stated that women should "take a lesson from men who have learned about the health dangers of their lifestyle. Give up smoking, quit eating and drinking to excess; and learn to go to the gym and exercise to reduce stress. For women, exercise is seen as just one more thing on their list of things to do. Learn to treat exercise as a reward. Learn that when you are under mental stress, doing something physical helps" (McIlhaney 1985, 687). Dr. Atkinson adds, "We must choose our priorities. We cannot be Super Woman."

Many women are trying to lead a Super Woman Lifestyle. Those who do not work outside the home are often involved in so many community, social, or child-related activities that they do not have time to take a deep breath. Women with careers are often trying to balance doing well on the job with being a good wife and mother, which obviously includes attending all the Little League games, piano recitals, and school performances in which their children participate.

These suggestions may be helpful in handling unproductive stress.

1. *Spend time alone.* Every woman needs some time just for herself. This is often neglected in our fast-paced world. Don't overextend yourself. Prioritize your activities so there is always time for "you."

2. *Spend time alone with your husband.* Every couple needs regular and uninterrupted time together to maintain an abiding relationship. Stresses within the marriage can often be improved by the increased communication that often develops from this kind of mutual sharing.

3. *Spend time with your family.* A woman who has family responsibilities but cannot find time to fulfill them adequately can feel a great deal of guilt and stress associated with this part of her life.

4. *Spend time with God.* There are some fantastic promises in the Bible to the person who develops a personal relationship with God. He helps us deal with the stresses of life as we learn to know and trust him.

5. *Avoid "stress eating."* What a vicious cycle! Look at this flow chart and see if it looks familiar:

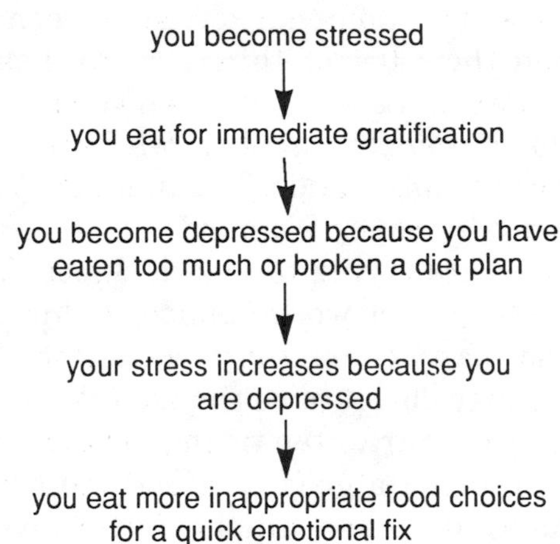
you become stressed
you eat for immediate gratification
you become depressed because you have eaten too much or broken a diet plan
your stress increases because you are depressed
you eat more inappropriate food choices for a quick emotional fix

This is called "a behavior chain" if it is something you do consistently. Many people react to stress in this way. It is in many ways very similar to tobacco or alcohol dependency in this situation. Break this cycle by "changing the subject." When you are tempted to snack, leave the situation—leave the house, leave the kitchen, do something like needlework with your hands, or go for a walk. Just do something different and try not to reinforce poor eating habits.

6. *Don't skip exercise time.* Endorphin release associated with aerobic exercise will give you a feeling of well-being and will absolutely help relieve stress. Don't skip it just because your schedule is tight and hectic. Exercise is an essential—not an extra.

7. *Prioritize your schedule.* Stress is often the result of overcommitment or poor time management—or both. Decide what is really important in your life and allow plenty of time for these activities.

8. *Consult specific books on stress control.* We suggest *Stress/Unstress* by Keith W. Sehnert (Minneapolis: Augsburg Publishing House, 1981); and *Living with Stress* by Lloyd H. Alhem (Ventura, Calif.: Regal Books, 1978).

9. *If things worsen . . .* you may need to consult your doctor, a psychiatrist or psychologist, or your pastor. Another source of help available in some communities is local workshops or clinics on stress. Expect expert assistance with stress problems from these sources. (See chapter 14 for more on this.)

Muscle Relaxation Techniques

Many people feel that taking a few minutes to slow down in the middle of the day is a great help in keeping daily stress under control. These exercises usually don't require more than fifteen minutes and can be especially useful in the afternoon or whenever your stress peaks. Though books have been written on muscle relaxation, the basic principles are really quite simple:

First, try to relax just your mind. Stop thinking about all those cares that came with today. Instead, you might concentrate on a favorite Scripture passage. Try to allow about twenty uninterrupted minutes in your bedroom or on the couch, somewhere that you will not be interrupted. A good tip is to take the phone off the hook.

Next, start relaxing your body, beginning with your toes. You should tense them, hold for the count of four, and then totally relax them. This exercise should be repeated all the way up your body: toes, feet and ankles, knees, thighs, buttocks, chest, arms, and finally your neck and shoulder area. Then just lie there for a few minutes—totally relaxed. Continue to chase any bad or worrisome thoughts away. Concentrate on the goodness of the Lord and the many blessings he has placed in your life.

14

Other Options

Counseling and PMS

The unfortunate long-term result of premenstrual syndrome can often be poor self-esteem and increasing difficulty with personal relationships. Even after physical PMS treatment has started and some of the symptoms are alleviated, the psychological scars of untreated PMS in years past can wreak havoc in peoples' lives. Depending on the severity of your psychological unrest, you or your physician may feel that some sort of counseling is in order. We strongly encourage you not to deny the potential usefulness of this important step in your complete treatment. Whether it is initially suggested by your physician, your husband, a friend, or was your own idea, be receptive and consider this option carefully.

First remember that approximately 50 percent of patients who see doctors about PMS do not actually have this syndrome. Other problems are creating the difficulty. If your problem is one of an emotional nature, it is extremely important that you see a psychiatrist, psychologist, or some other counselor. Have your problems assessed correctly. If you and your physician cannot be sure whether psychological problems are the basis for what seems to be PMS, it may be important for you to have psychological testing done. We would encourage you to take those tests if they are suggested.

It is sometimes difficult to know with whom to start your counseling. If you prefer Christian-oriented counseling and your personal physician is a Christian, he or she can probably direct you to a Christian psychologist (with a master's degree or doctorate in psychology), a Christian psychiatrist (an M.D. with specialized training after medical school in the area of clinical psychiatry), or a Christian counselor (probably with a strong background in psychology and training in counseling).

If your physician is not able to provide such references, you might seek advice from your minister. (Some churches allow their ministers time for counseling members, and pastoral counseling might be a good choice if other options are financially out of the question.) If you need counseling and are a Christian, we strongly suggest that you seek a like-minded counselor. A Christian counselor will understand your life philosophy and value system, will be able to pray with you, and will work with you toward spiritual growth as you heal emotionally.

Hysterectomy as a "Solution" to PMS

Patients who have a great deal of trouble controlling their PMS or who cannot control it will often ask their physicians about having a hysterectomy to correct their problem. Hysterectomy may or may not stop the PMS problems, which is why a doctor who agrees that a hysterectomy is an appropriate course of action may suggest removing the ovaries at the time of the hysterectomy. This procedure will eliminate PMS problems in many women, but is still not 100 percent effective. There are some patients who still have some PMS symptoms, even when the uterus, ovaries, and tubes are removed. No one understands how this can happen, but apparently the brain's hypothalamus produces a pattern that causes monthly body cycles, which a few women can feel even with their uterus, tubes, and ovaries removed.

A decision for this type of major surgery should not be made hastily. It is a decision that should be carefully discussed with your physician and appropriate family members. It goes without saying that it should not be done until you reach the point in your life where the birth of additional children is totally undesired. If you do decide to have a hysterectomy, we recommend that you also have your ovaries removed. That procedure will give you the greatest chance for relief of your PMS symptoms.

If you do have your uterus, tubes, and ovaries removed for relief of PMS, you must then take estrogen if you are below the age of forty-five (I advise my patients to take estrogen even if they are older than forty-five). Estrogen will prevent the development of osteoporosis and will decrease the chance of developing heart disease later.

I would recommend that a woman who has had a hysterectomy for PMS not take progesterone after her surgery: (1) because most doctors do not think it is necessary (and I agree); (2) also since PMS seems in some ways caused by progesterone, or at least by the progesterone phase of the cycle, that phase can be eliminated after the removal of a woman's uterus, tubes, and ovaries, simply by her not taking progesterone. The natural form of progesterone may be used later if there seems to be need for such medication.

PMS Clinics

There are a number of specialized PMS clinics around the country. The primary advantage of these clinics is that if you choose to go to one, you can be assured of seeing health-care specialists who are interested in PMS and its treatment. However, if you can find an interested private physician (preferably an obstetrician/gynecologist or family practitioner) you can usually get equally good care in what may be a more personal environment. It is also generally easier to maintain an ongoing, long-term relationship with a private physician than with a more impersonal clinic.

The staff at PMS clinics usually consists of a nurse practitioner, a health educator, a psychologist, an obstetrics/gynecology physician, a physical therapist, a dietitian, and sometimes a marriage therapist and social worker. You will normally pay several hundred dollars for evaluation and treatment. These clinics generally give good care for women with PMS.

If you prefer going to your own physician for PMS, he or she can refer you to the other health professionals listed above to complete your treatment program if it seems to be necessary.

One way you might use a PMS clinic, even if you do not want to be treated there as a patient, is to call and ask which private physicians in your area they recommend for the treatment of PMS. Be aware, however, that these clinics are "for profit" organizations and may imply that no one else in the geographic area can help you as much as they can. This may or may not be true.

Support Groups

If you live in a larger metropolitan area, there may be a local support group for PMS sufferers. The only nationwide support group we are aware of is:

PMS Access
P.O. Box 9326
Madison, WI 53715

Phone: 1-800-222-4PMS

Since this is a division of the Madison Pharmacy Associates, they will probably want to sell you books and other PMS materials. However, they seem reputable and, for the most part, their information appears to be accurate and reliable.

15

Your Spiritual Life and PMS

The Spiritual Dilemma

Many Christian women who have PMS feel guilty because of their recurring behavior patterns—anger, depression, irritability—during their PMS cycle. Such women feel that they are not in a right relationship with God when these reactions occur, because such behaviors do not reflect a close walk with God. These women, and you may be one of them, will often be loving, caring, God-obeying women the rest of the month, but when the PMS cycle occurs, they seem to no longer exhibit the fruit of the Spirit. Often they become guilt-ridden about this.

To such women we have a loud and clear message: *PMS is not a spiritual problem!* The anger, resentment, depression, and so on, are a result of physical changes in a woman's body. When a woman feels this way she is not guilty of being out of fellowship with God every month during her PMS time, even though she may feel she is. For example, if your husband stays up all night tonight, all day tomorrow, and all tomorrow night, he will probably be tired, irritable, and short-tempered by the next day, not because he is out of fellowship with God but because his physical body does not feel well. It is tired. A woman with

PMS who does not have any abiding separation from God will feel many negative emotions, not because of a spiritual problem but because her body does not feel well during PMS time.

Christian women who can grasp this truth can shed a great deal of guilt. They can then get on with the task of doing those things necessary to minimize their PMS symptoms.

When the husband of a woman with PMS understands that PMS behavior is caused by physical changes in her body and not because she is spiritually weak or because Satan has a hold on her, the husband can get on with the job of helping his wife overcome PMS. If your husband does not seem to understand, encourage him to read this book, especially the sections written specifically to husbands in the introduction and in chapter 12. That may help him to become a partner with you in overcoming PMS.

We are not saying that God is not involved with a woman who has PMS. We believe that God can totally take away a woman's PMS just as he can miraculously heal a woman of breast cancer. However, it seems that the more usual way he works in a woman's life is to enable her to have the desire and discipline to take the medical steps necessary for overcoming PMS.

If a woman has unresolved guilt, a heart filled with anger that she refuses to release, and so on, her spiritual problem can make the PMS time even worse. We encourage all women to look objectively at their relationship with God, confess any known sin, and then not blame themselves for the monthly changes that are definitely PMS-related but can so cleverly mimic spiritual weakness.

Prayer and PMS

All of life's situations need prayer, and this includes PMS. During the PMS time, you may feel that God doesn't hear your prayers and is far from you. In fact, he hears and is close, as always. Prayer is a tremendous tool. Pray often and pray in faith. When you pray with regard to your PMS, you might keep these things in mind:

1. *Pray regularly.* Be sure to continue your prayers and fellowship with God when you are premenstrual. This may seem unnatural at first, especially before the treatment program takes effect. Many women feel out of fellowship at this time and thus avoid prayer time. Don't fall into this trap.
2. *Pray for the right physician.* Pray that God will lead you to a physician who will meet your own needs.
3. *Pray for a treatment program* that will free you from PMS problems.
4. *Pray for perseverance in your treatment program.* Pray that God will give you the inner strength to continue your treatment program indefinitely. This includes careful attention to diet and exercise.
5. *Pray for your family and friends.* Pray that with education and acceptance, your loved ones can come to understand this problem more clearly.

Bibliography

Abraham, G. E. "Nutritional Factors in the Etiology of the Premenstrual Syndrome." *The Journal of Reproductive Medicine* 28 (1983): 446.

———— and R. E. Rumley. "Role of Nutrition in Managing the Premenstrual Tension Syndromes." *Journal of Reproductive Medicine* 32 (1987): 405–422.

Barber, H. R. *The Female Patient* (October, 1986): 9–16.

Boyle, C. A., G. Berkowitz and J. Kelsey. "Epidemiology of Premenstrual Syndrome." *American Journal of Public Health* 77 (1987): 349–350.

Brayshaw, Nora. *American Health* 417 (1985): 76.

Chihal, H. Jane. *Clinical Review* 21 (1981): 99.

————. *Premenstrual Syndrome: A Clinic Manual.* Durant, Okla.: Creative Informatics, Inc., 1985.

Crook, W. *The Yeast Connection.* Jackson, Tenn.: Professional Books of Future Health, Inc., 1985.

Dalton, K. *The Premenstrual Syndrome and Progesterone Therapy.* London: Heinemann Medical Books, Ltd., 1984.

Dawood, M., J. McGuire, M. Laurence, *Premenstrual Syndrome and Dysmenorrhea.* Baltimore:Urban and Schwarzenberg, 1985.

Frank, R. T. *Archives of Neurologic Psychiatry* 26 (1931): 1053–1057.

Gannon, L. *Menstrual Disorders and Menopause.* Baltimore: Praeger, 1985.

Grant, J. P. *Handbook of Total Parenteral Nutrition.* Philadelphia: W. B. Saunders, 1980.

Gregory, B. A. *Journal of Psychosomatic Research* 2 (1957): 61–79.

Harrison, M. *Self-help for Premenstrual Syndrome.* New York: Random House, 1985.

Holmes, T. J. and R. H. Rabe. *Journal of Psychosomatic Research* 11 (1967).

Johnson, S. R. *Clinical Obstetrics and Gynecology* 30 (1987): 367.

Kantero, R. L. and C. Widholm. *Acta Obstetrica Gynecologia Scandinavia* 14 (1971): 17–18.

McIlhaney, J. and S. Nethery. *1250 Health-Care Questions Women Ask.* Grand Rapids, Michigan: Baker Book House, 1985.

Mortola, J. F. *OB/GYN News* April (1987).

Norris, R. V. *Premenstrual Syndrome.* New York: Berkeley Books, 1984.

Pennington, V. M. *Journal of the American Medical Association* 638 (1957): 164.

Prior, J. C., Y. Vigna and N. Alojada. *European Journal of Applied Physiology* 55 (1986): 349–355.

Rogers, F. S. *American Journal of Obstetrics and Gynecology* 59 (1950): 321–327.

Trobisch, I. *The Joy of Being A Woman.* New York: Harper and Row, 1975.

van den Berg, H., E. S. Louwerse, H. W. Bruinse, J. T. Thissen, and J. Schrijver. "Vitamin B_6 Status of Women Suffering from Premenstrual Syndrome." Human Nutrition: Clinical Nutrition 40C (1986): 441–450.

Van Regenmorter, J., S. van Regenmorter, and J. McIlhaney, *Dear God, Why Can't We Have a Baby?* Grand Rapids, Michigan: Baker Book House, 1986.

Vellacott, A. and C. O'Brien. *Journal of Reproductive Medicine* 32 (1987): 429.

Index